"Dee's book is insightf[ul] fantastic source of info[r] who support them. Sha[re] amputee herself, Dee il[lustrates] loss of a limb is a challe[nge]

Dan Broome, Above knee amputation from trauma, Project Manager for Grading & Demolition Co., California, Member US Amputee Soccer Team.

"With clarity, wit and an accessible style, limb salvage specialist Dee Malchow (herself a high-functioning lower extremity amputee) provides a "how-to" guide for patients (and their families) confronted by the possibility -- or the established fact -- of limb loss. As an amputation surgeon myself for the past 40 years, how I wish I had had available this handbook to help educate, calm, reassure and (believe it or not) even amuse my amputation patients! Kudos to Dee Malchow for providing absolutely essential insight into this terribly fraught clinical scenario."

Kaj Johansen MD, PhD, FACS, Chief of Vascular Surgery at Swedish Medical Center, Seattle

"Alive and Whole, Amputation: Emotional Recovery by Dee Malchow, is an excellent book. It is a comprehensive self-help book that is well organized and easy to read. The information will benefit anyone, and everyone, who must deal with amputation and/or other major losses. It was an honor to work with Ms. Malchow on this project."

Crystal Linn, literary consultant, Amazon top-selling author

"I have just read this book with great enjoyment and interest. It brought back a flood of great memories, as I was a colleague of

Dee throughout her time at Harborview. She helped me perfect a diurnal pain medication regime which kept patients asleep at night and awake and interacting in the daytime. I also came to realize she was spending extra time counseling new amputee patients at night. We conceived the idea of an amputee clinic and support group with her as the leader. The hospital administration soon realized the value of Dee's program and 'the rest is history…' as they say.

Everyone who deals in any way with patients who have incurred a disfiguring and/or disabling injury will find reading this book time very well spent."

Sig T. Hansen Jr. MD, Professor Emeritus, University of Washington, School of Medicine; Director of Sigvard T. Hansen Foot & Ankle Institute, Harborview Medical Center, Seattle.

"I was given this book to review from an author friend who wanted my perspective having been in the military for twenty years and currently working in law enforcement. Dee Malchow has written a very easy to read and easy to understand book dealing with amputation. This book covers everything for the experience of first losing a limb, grief, acceptance and even things I wouldn't have imagined, like families reactions, phantom feelings and intimacy.

I have dealt with plenty of amputees in my careers, but after reading Dee's book, I have a whole new understanding of what someone who has been through this type of loss may or may not be going through. I highly recommend this book to anyone whether you work in a field where you deal with this or not. This book was an eye opener for me, something I never truly looked at or perhaps, didn't want to look at."

William Tasch, Amazon best-selling author

Alive and Whole

Amputation: Emotional Recovery

Dee Malchow MN, RN

Copyright © 2015 Dee Malchow

All rights reserved.

ISBN: **1622085582**
ISBN-13: **978-1622085583**

DEDICATION

To the people who live with an amputation and

those who love them.

.

CONTENTS

Table of Contents

Acknowledgements

Forward

Chapter 1 --- My First Encounter	19
Chapter 2 --- Grief Reaction	25
Shock	26
Denial	28
Grief	29
Anger	30
Anxiety	31
Chapter 3 --- Acceptance	34
Our Attitude	35
The 'Super Amputee'	37
Need to Prove Something	38
Identity	39
Risky Behavior	40
Mental Health Issues	41
Chapter 4 --- Adjustment	43
Home	43
Driving	44
Work	45
Play	46
Camaraderie	48
Internet	49
Legal Issues	49
Chapter 5 --- Saving a Limb	51

Parents	51
Patient	52
Doctor	52
Survival	52
Body Preservation	53
Saving the Unsaveable	54
Doctors' Struggle	55
Ultimate Cost	57
Chapter 6 --- Reactions of Family, Friends and Others	**59**
Other People with Amputations	61
Others' Reactions	61
Humor	62
Negative Reactions	63
Prejudice	64
Dissupport	64
Supporters Need Support Too	66
Impact on Family	66
Chapter 7 --- Spiritual Concerns	**68**
Personal Experience	69
Other Faiths	70
Death	70
Anger	71
Evaluation	72
Chapter 8 --- Body Image and Sexuality	**73**
Self-Esteem	74

Feelings about Sexuality	76
Devotees	79
Chapter 9 --- Socio-Cultural Implications	81
Pity	81
Shame	82
Uselessness	82
Criminal	83
Cursed	83
Marriageability	84
Changing Biases	85
Our Part	86
Chapter 10 -- Feelings about Pain	87
Duration	87
Degrees of Pain	87
Drug Dependence	88
Pain Following Surgery	89
Becoming a Survivor	90
Chapter 11 -- Phantom Feelings	92
Phantom	94
Chapter 12 -- Doctors Have Feelings Too	96
Salvage Preferred	96
Destructive vs. Reconstructive	97
Quality of Life	98
Emotional Connection	99
Hard Cases	100
Chapter 13 – Money – The Bottom Line	102
Home Management and Care of Others	102

Insurance	102
Cost to Family	103
Employment	103
Professional Performers	105
Chapter 14 -- Feelings about My Prosthesis	107
Disappointment	107
Prosthetist	108
The First Prosthetic	108
Reality	109
Clothing Alterations	110
Comfort and Feel	112
Reliability	113
Safety	114
Ongoing Adjustment	115
Chapter 15 -- Summary of Coping with	
Limb Loss	118
Grief	118
Support System	118
Support Group	119
Information	119
Rebuilding Physically	120
Think Positive	121
Humor	122
Utilize Necessary Available Benefits	123
Avoid Extensive Drug Use and Self-Pity	125

Reach Out to Others	125

Appendix -

Dealing with Loss	128
Helping Others with Loss	130
Footstone (an amputation poem)	132
Glossary	133
End Notes	135

Acknowledgements

It is with much gratitude that I acknowledge the many people who live with amputations that have shared their hearts, minds and souls with me over the years. Besides the good Lord, they are my true inspiration for this book.

My special tribute goes to Crystal Linn who has kindly and patiently mentored me through this writing. She has helped me with my technology challenges as well as served as a valuable editor throughout. Thank you also to Ray Rupert, who initially directed me to Crystal and to Helping Hands Press, my publisher.

Over the years I have worked alongside several amazing physicians who constantly demonstrate special caring for their patients who experience limb loss. Among these are Dr. Doug G. Smith, Dr. Sigvard T. Hansen, and Dr Kaj Johansen. They taught me much about the doctors' view of amputations, and so much more. I thank them for taking the time to review this book and giving helpful feedback and encouragement.

A special prayer team has kept me on task as they provided encouragement through prayer and enthusiastic words. They include Jessica Ruble, Sue MacFarlane, Julie Tiersma, Carol Helt, and Crystal Linn. Others have also prayed for me and I am grateful for them as well. You have each been more vital than you realize in the writing of this manuscript.

Dee Malchow MN, RN

Shoreline, Washington

September, 2014

Forward

As a nurse with an amputation specializing in the care of amputees, I am often confronted with the question from trembling lips, "The doctor says I need an amputation. How do people make that work? Or do they?"

The answers to these questions are varied, and quite extensive. So I decided to answer these and other questions in this book.

When I began to write, it became clear that this information could be useful to people dealing with limb loss and many other losses as well. We all live a life that will eventually encounter loss. Perhaps it will be a death, loss of a home, job, marriage or other precious relationship. It ultimately threatens our dreams and plans for the future. My desire is to help soften the loss, encourage the survivor and give hope.

Since becoming an amputee myself over fifty years ago, I have had the privilege of interacting with more than 3,000 amputees. This has occurred primarily through my job as an orthopedic nurse. It expanded further when I became a clinical nurse specialist in the field of amputation care. In that role I served as coordinator of the Limb Viability Service at Harborview, Seattle's Level I Trauma Center. This service provides assistance with decision making for those who may lose or have lost a limb. It also provides health care networking connections for the best surgery, therapy and rehabilitation.

My exposure to people with amputations was expanded through involvement in amputee skiing and soccer programs. Research in artificial limbs (prosthetics) gave me an added group of people to interact with. Most recently I've participated in mission outreach to the amputees of the recovering, war torn nation of Sierra Leone in

West Africa. These unique encounters affirmed that I should put in writing some of the first-hand knowledge gained about this fascinating population that I belong to.

My personal experiences are sprinkled throughout. The first chapter contains the story of my intimate introduction to the amputee population, when I became one. In some ways this book is 'my story', but it is much more than that. It includes multiple experiences and comments made by people with amputations that I have encountered. There is some reference to other published literature related to this subject. This is all combined with my added education in psychology and personal adjustment process. For reasons of privacy, real names are not used except as stated otherwise.

There is minimal discussion on the technical aspects of surgery, rehabilitation and prosthetics. The emotions of the amputee, and those close to them, are the focus of this book.

There is also discussion of the feelings of those who must do the amputating – the surgeons. Essentially, 'how do people feel about having a limb removed and how do the people feel who have to do the removing?'

This book is written to provide information. Ideally it will give hope and encouragement to the individual who is facing an amputation, as well as those who have already survived one. Some of us had no opportunity to prepare for the event. Even those who saw it coming never seem quite 'ready' for it. Ultimately, it is my desire that this book will be a useful tool for a healthy recovery in the hands of the person facing an amputation as well as the new amputee. Perhaps it can even help the person who has lived many years with an amputation sort out some old emotions that never came together well in the past.

Amputation is life changing and has a profound impact on all those around us. Therefore, I further desire that this information will assist family, friends, health care professionals, and society in general, to understand the experience better. It is anticipated that many people who have dealt with issues of loss, at every level, will relate easily to the emotions and adjustment processes discussed herein.

For purposes of readability, the amputee will be referred to as 'him' throughout this book except in specific instances dealing with females. This is to avoid the cumbersome his/her pronoun reference. It is also sensible since amputees are often males. Females account for less than twenty percent of traumatic amputations.

My preference is to refer to an amputee as a 'person with an amputation' (which is what we are). We are first and foremost, a person. Each of us is so much more than that one factor of our body or identity. However, for simplicity and clarity I've chosen to stick with the generic descriptive word 'amputee' in many places. I trust this will not be offensive to my readers.

Finally, the latter portion of the book is meant to tie it all together. It is a summary of the things to do and not do in order to make our lives incorporate our significant loss and move forward.

1 MY FIRST ENCOUNTER

As the boat rapidly approached me on the windswept water of the murky, secluded lake I was about to have my first encounter with an amputee…myself.

Water skiing was something I had never tried. When two other nursing students suggested we take a break from studying for this venture, I was game. It was a delightfully warm mid-July evening in 1964. A construction worker at the hospital, Perry, and his cousin, Al, had a boat. They invited us to join them for some water skiing. So we headed to a small lake just south of Wenatchee, a town in central Washington.

Tammy and I had almost completed our first year of nurses' education. The other student was Holly, who was nearly finished with her full three years of the program. We were in a small 'diploma' nursing school (only thirty-six students) affiliated with the main hospital in the beautiful orchard country of the Wenatchee Valley, in Washington State.

It happened so quickly. After falling off the water skis twice I then awaited my friends who were in the boat, as they picked up and brought one of the errant skis back to me. Suddenly I realized that the boat was coming much too fast. Perry was driving his cousin's boat. When he saw that he was coming at me too fast, he turned abruptly to the left. But the wind and boat speed robbed him of control. In the meantime I had turned in the water and was vigorously attempting to swim to the right and away from his panicky skid. The bulky life vest I wore encumbered my efforts as I kicked to get away. Then I felt the prop hit with a significant thud. The propeller grabbed and sliced my right leg completely up the back before the boat spun away with its horrified cargo.

I bobbed like a cork in the eerie silence of the aftermath. As I attempted to kick again, the pain struck suddenly and fiercely. I screamed for help as the most unbearable pain I have ever known, before or since, overtook me.

The boat appeared quickly alongside me. My friends worked together to lift me gently out of the water as they gasped at the sight before them. The intense pain and their verbal reaction conveyed to me that I might never see this extremity again.

As I stole a brief look at my right leg, I looked almost as quickly away, as a wave of nausea rolled silently over me. *Surely it will drop off at any minute*, I thought, *perhaps before we get to the hospital.* But it didn't. I couldn't process the enormity of it all, either physically or emotionally. I was in shock. I was hoping to simply pass out, but I didn't.

Lying there in the boat in a pool of my own blood, I thought of crying or screaming as the agonizing pain continued relentlessly. But I had no strength for that. *Besides*, I thought, *why bother? My friends are doing what they can to care for me and get me rapidly to the hospital.* Strangely, underneath it all, I didn't want to further upset them. That's how we nurses tend to think – lots of empathy for others.

How grateful I felt for the two student-nurse friends with me who rapidly applied their first aid training. They first wrapped towels firmly around my leg to slow some of the bleeding. I was not surprised when Holly, the senior student, said they needed a tourniquet. She found a belt and applied it quickly to my right upper thigh.

A tourniquet, we had just been taught, was only to be used when survival was the issue. It surely would threaten even further, the life of my leg. The profound implications of this act struck me but I quickly released the thought. There was no time or energy to ponder it. I needed to survive and endure the pain for now. What was happening so quickly was too great to process. Just staying alive was my job.

I felt weak as I lay there talking audibly to God. "Please help me, Jesus. I love you." My faith is a relationship with God as my loving Father. It is close and personal. I speak often to Him and His Son, Jesus, each day – especially during any crisis.

Breathing became laborious as my lifeblood drained out slowly and coagulated in the boat bottom. I considered death as it loomed like a dark gray cloud before me.

I had entrusted my life and my soul to Jesus as a child. I was forgiven and loved by my Creator. I felt safe and peaceful in that knowledge. *But, Lord*, I prayed, silently in the boat, *I don't want to leave here yet*. So much of my life had not been lived. My subconscious dreams of what the future might hold gave a sense of reluctance at the thought of death. *What about marriage, children, becoming a nurse...?*

The boat was driven quickly onto the shore. As Al held the bow of the boat Perry ran to a house across the road to call for help. It seemed much too long as we awaited the ambulance in that rural setting. Finally we heard it in a distance – the beautiful wail of a siren. *Thank you, Lord.*

The attendants carefully lifted me onto a stretcher but the searing pain was magnified by every move. I groaned loudly as they spoke apologetically and carefully loaded me into the ambulance. My student nurse friends scrambled in as the attendant placed a mask over my face and began administering oxygen to my deprived lungs. Ah-h-h, it tasted like fresh air in stuffy room. It was much easier to breathe. A glance to my left showed that the young attendant was the same cute guy who had helped teach our first aid class last week. *Rats*, I thought momentarily, w*hat a way to get to meet him.*

I felt every excruciating bump as the driver moved as smoothly as he could over the rocky dirt driveway from the lake to the pavement. At last we were on the move as the sirens wailed outside. My friends told me later that there were two vehicles - our ambulance and a police car ahead of us. Our speed moved up to ninety-five miles per hour. A brief thought went through my mind. *Too bad I don't get to enjoy this ride.* I'd never ridden in an emergency vehicle before.

The hospital arrival was as I had hoped. Pain relief at last. So much was happening as they were trying to contact my parents and order some blood to replace my loss. I quickly announced that I knew my blood type to be O Positive, thinking that would expedite everything. The doctor politely informed me that my blood needed to be cross matched with other factors anyway, as the nurse slid the needle into my arm. Well, phooey! Knowing my blood type had seemed like important information for such an emergency. But nobody really cared. In my state of shock and injury, I don't think they would have taken my word for it anyway.

Once I was comfortable from the spinal anesthetic, the emergency room nurses began to prepare me for the operating room. My bathing suit needed to be removed. Scissors were picked up as they gently informed me of this next step.

"No." I pleaded. It was a one-piece suit with a lovely pink flowered print. "I just got it new and I really like it. Can't we just take it off some other way?" They were kind but insistent that it needed to be removed this way and couldn't be saved. And so began the losses that went along with this tragic injury.

The medical team worked most of the night piecing my leg back together. There was now no pain but I could hear the tapping and feel the jarring as they put a rod down the bone to connect the five breaks in my lower leg. Occasionally I would arouse and talk with the staff that was familiar to me in the small hospital. At one point I remember asking if I could look at my leg as they worked on it. The anesthetist said that wouldn't be a good idea. I tried to press the issue and very soon I slipped away into a deep sleep. Ha, he had the upper hand on that one.

Hundreds of stitches later I was finally wheeled into the recovery room. Glancing down at my leg, I saw my toes sticking out of a cast that was propped on a pillow. *Huh?*, I thought, *my leg is just badly broken? Perhaps things are not as bad as they seemed at first.*

As I was wheeled to my room, I saw my dad, mom and brother in the waiting area. I was genuinely surprised as I commented, "What are you guys doing here?" They had driven slightly above the speed limit, I later learned, from our home north of Seattle. I guess I would expect them at some time but not the middle of the night for 'just a broken leg'.

Perry was also sitting in the waiting area, looking like the proverbial 'basket case'. Compassion overwhelmed me as I saw the guilt of his carelessness hanging visibly on his shoulders. The thought crossed my mind, *I'm glad I'm me and not him. I'd hate to know that I'd done this to someone.* I wasn't angry at him. It was an accident.

In the nursing dormitory across the street another doctor had checked on the students. Tammy was pretty upset and was given a sedative to sleep. She wasn't sure if I would make it through the night. I also believe the visuals of the accident were harder on her while my eyes were closed most of the time. A couple weeks later Tammy went to a Disney adventure movie where someone in the water was being pursued by a motorboat. She screamed and left the theater.

The next few days were unclear to me as a fever took over and I thrashed to find comfort. While the world focused on things like Viet Nam, race riots, and the Beatles, I prayed vigorously for my badly damaged leg. In the fog of my fever, I saw a variety of doctors come by looking seriously at my immobile, dusky toes. My student nurse friends were often around. They quietly tried to make me comfortable and make nutritious milkshakes and other concoctions that I might drink. I wasn't too interested but made efforts to drink them knowing that I needed to get well.

Three days after the injury the heroic battle to save my leg was surrendered to the white flag of survival. Gangrene had set in along with the vicious bacteria called pseudomonas. The threat to my life was traded rapidly for the high price of my lower right leg. Although the propeller had sliced deeply in nine places up to my hip, Sovereign control and skilled surgical intervention salvaged my right knee and resulted in an amputation about three and one-half inches below it.

This time, as I revived momentarily in the recovery room, I raised my head and glanced briefly at my right lower extremity. No foot or leg lifted the sheet in the natural form that had been there for 19 years. It was flat…empty. I rested my head back on the pillow with great sadness but also an odd sense of relief. *It's over*, I breathed silently. But it had only begun…

2 GRIEF REACTION

Most people who have a missing limb were not born that way. They were forced, like me, to experience a dramatic change to their body. Along with the physical loss, we were forced to deal with the accompanying emotional impact of that loss. Those who have lived with limb loss since birth still have a physical difference to deal with. Not a change, but a difference. They also experience a lifetime of dealing with people's reaction to that loss.

Of the estimated two million amputees in the United States, less than 3 percent entered life without their limb(s). The majority of amputations, about 82 percent, result from limited blood circulation (blood vessel disease and/or diabetes). Trauma or injury cause about 12 percent and cancer accounts for the balance of all amputations.[i]

As with any severe loss, there are emotional stages of recovery.[ii] The person with the amputation attempts to determine how or even if he can survive. There are differing opinions on the process, but there are common emotional phases a person may encounter. These may include shock, denial, bargaining, anger, grief, anxiety and acceptance/adjustment. For now I want to discuss the first six probable phases. The following chapters will deal more extensively with acceptance and adjustment.

Not everyone goes through each stage, nor do they always

follow a rigid sequence. Experiencing some of the emotional phases seems to allow our whole being the opportunity to recover and regroup from life changing losses like an amputation. It allows us the opportunity to move forward.

Getting stuck in any stage is always a possibility. Reality and positive connections from those who care about us are a part of what pushes us on. I see that the leg is gone. My family encourages me and smiles with enthusiasm as I take my first step on crutches. I want to move forward for myself and for them so I choose not to give up in my hard situation.

Shock

The reality of the loss is there in front of us as a new amputee. Our mind may be screaming, *No, it's all a bad dream! I can't believe it!* But there it is. The emotional shock and denial attempt to protect us from this awful reality. However, the image of the shortened extremity is ever before us; first in vision, then by touch, and immediately in loss of function. We see it's not there, we feel the shortened limb, and we stop suddenly as we attempt to do one of the many tasks this extremity used to do. Unlike the new paralytic who may say in protective denial, *"I walked yesterday and I'll walk again tomorrow."* the new amputee is missing a crucial body part. It can't just be talked into existence. Function, obviously, is gone with the body part, at least temporarily.

Reality, to some extent, begins to settle in after surgery. It begins with the 'flat sheet' on the affected side or the otherwise conspicuous absence of the extremity. As described previously, this was my own experience as well.

I heard another person say, "I looked down at the bed and the sheet was flat where my foot and leg used to be. There was no need to look under it."

The amputee's arm or leg is not occupying the space in proximity to the body that it once did. Except for the strange phantom sensation (which will be discussed in detail later), we become acutely aware from sight, touch, and feedback from others that the extremity is no longer a part of our body. At first it seems like only a cold, impersonal piece of information.

This harsh fact may hit us early. One man said, "I knew immediately that my hand was gone," as he and his mangled hand were lifted from beneath the forklift.

Another lady said, "When the bus ran over my foot, it looked like hamburger. I knew it couldn't be saved." It's an immediate fact; we observe but cannot include full comprehension of all that lies ahead.

One day soon after surgery the bandage or cast over the wound is removed. There, underneath it all is the surgically revised limb, or, as one lady said, "What was left of it and what wasn't."

Stark reality jumps out at the amputee as our limb is viewed, touched, moved and felt in a new and often frighteningly strange way. This odd appendage is a part of our body now. At best it looks like a shortened version of the old limb without a hand or foot on the end. At worst, it is bizarrely scarred and misshapen. There may be no resemblance to a human body – much less the familiar part that used to function from this extremity for so many years. In the beginning, mine was swollen on the end, making it look like a club. The shortened leg was totally unattractive and almost repulsive.

One lady confided, "It looked so ugly. I was glad that the doctor said it looked good and was healing well. Nothing looked good about it to me!"

Emotional shock may go on for several days, or even weeks, as we focus on recovery from the impact of whatever caused the loss. There is a struggle to physically survive and carry on with basic body functions (breathing, drinking, eating, sleeping, etc.).Thoughts about the loss are often pushed aside as we sink under the load of drugs, surgery and exhaustion.

A classic example of shock is Scarlett O'Hara in the movie and book, <u>Gone with the Wind</u>, numbly stating, "I'll think about that tomorrow." Her beloved plantation, Tara, is burning down.[iii] There's just too much to process all at once.

Denial

Denial, as mentioned previously, may be presumed to not exist at all. "I accepted it from the beginning," one man said, "my leg was gone and that was that!" As his nurse, I was not convinced, but said nothing. He was willing to accept a fact but it was far too soon to accept, or even know, how his life will be impacted by this loss.

The defense mechanism of denial is typically present and can be of great value. The eyes of the amputee send a clear message to the brain, "*This is real, something is missing.*" That reality is only comprehended in part. The limb may be gone but what does that mean to his life? If it's a leg, he can't even get up and walk to the bathroom. If it's an arm, he can't tie the string on the back of his hospital gown or open the milk carton on his meal tray. Denial slides steadily into grief as the awareness of these and more limits and more fears settle in.

His natural jumble of thoughts may include, *Will people reject me? Will I lose my job? Can my girlfriend handle this? Can I continue to play my favorite sport? Do I want to live like this? Can I?*

Nearly all amputees experience significant emotions when the cast or bandage is first removed. The 'damage' is now out in the open for the owner of the limb and everyone there to see. It's hard (impossible?) to deny the reality of his loss at this point.

The gauze bandage seems to sometimes soften the emotional impact of the first viewing. The person has been able to identify with the humanity of the altered limb by moving, touching and feeling its warmth. However, the first vision of the body part under it all is still disturbing in most cases. The process of claiming ownership of this strange unfamiliar extremity usually begins when viewed 'in the flesh'. It takes time to get acquainted with one's own body in this new altered state.

Reality seems to be shielded even more effectively if a cast is put on the shortened limb in the operating room right after surgery. The cast may stay in place for several days, making it easier to cling to a type of denial. This is especially so if a temporary leg and foot is attached to the bottom of the cast. The person can put it all under the sheet for a short while and speak abstractly about the 'injury' or 'surgery'.

It may be that the individual prefers to delay viewing his changed limb. Denial can protect and defend the ego for a while longer. Viewing it may be best postponed for a later date and a safer place, like home. Then, if emotion arises, it can be expressed without having to pretend strength and acceptance for the benefit of the health care personnel and others present. Some have approached this 'getting acquainted' process in steps.

First they listen to what the doctor says following examination. Then a trusted family member or friend views it and describes it to him. Some have even had photos taken of the healing extremity and looked at them carefully first. Everyone has their own approach.

Most people, however, are overcome by curiosity and look at their limb as soon as the opportunity arises. Unfortunately, the altered extremity will be there for a long while. Early viewing is not necessary and does not, in my professional experience, correlate with the degree of ultimate acceptance of the loss. This is usually a difficult event. Looking at the revised limb later may even result in more preparation and less negative feelings about the looks of it.

Grief

Some new amputees wait until they get home to deal with the grief. It's usually a safer haven in which to say what they feel and express their pain. Most can't wait that long, however, and will express some strong emotion when denial has lifted and left reality in its place. The emotional load may be expressed in tears, anger, and/or withdrawal.

For me, the tears of grief came immediately after the doctor left the room with the news that my leg had to be removed that very afternoon. There had been three days for me to ponder the implications of purple numb toes, a raging fever, and the sober faces of the medical consultants examining my leg.

When I finished crying, Sue, my student nurse friend asked if she could do anything. I asked her to read my Bible to me, from the book of Romans. The words gave me a sense of peace and solace as I collapsed back on the pillow. A couple times I cried late at night to release the deep pain in my heart. The hard knot in my stomach and lump in my throat seemed to relax with the tears.

Many people have told me that they cried in the intensive care unit as they began to comprehend what had happened. One man admitted, "When I asked her, the nurse told me that my leg was gone. I cried for a little while."

Some said that seeing family or friends in the beginning triggered great emotion. One young man who had lost both legs under a train said, "I was doing ok but then when mom walked into the room I couldn't hold it back. We both just bawled and hugged each other."

Anger

Some people feel more anger than sadness. Typical comments are, "It's not fair! Why me?", "Why was I (or someone else) so stupid and careless?", "The doctors didn't try hard enough to save it.", "When I get out of here I'm going to get the drunk that caused this!", "I'm going to sue (whomever) for all they've got!" The emotion seems to depend on personality as well as the circumstances of the loss. Some people just automatically get mad when something goes wrong in their life.

One young man from Alaska lost his leg while apparently driving recklessly. He was asked how he normally dealt with hard stuff in his life. He honestly replied as he gritted his teeth, "I usually go down to the bar and knock a few heads around."

Psychologists say that people are inclined to either turn their emotions inward on themselves or outward on others. People who turn inward express sadness with a loss and those who turn outward get angry. Fortunately, an amputation does not usually result in extreme actions even though a myriad of intense thoughts typically occur in the beginning. Many of the amputees I've talked with have shared the honest initial thought, "I'd rather be dead than live like this."

Professional help should be sought if vengeful anger is extreme or disabling sadness continues for a long period. Ongoing thoughts or specific plans of suicide must also be taken seriously. The medical team and family need to be alert to when added support is called for.

Anxiety

Expressions of grief in some form are often followed by anxious thoughts about the future. "Now that I've vented, cried, talked, screamed, or moped, about all this - what am I going to do about it?" If he's typical, he's never faced anything quite like this before and he doesn't really know anyone personally who has.

On a rare occasion a new amputee will have had previous contact with an experienced amputee. But this is uncommon. Perhaps a relative or a friend has had a limb loss. If so, a lot will depend on how well that person did with it. One woman said, with great fear in her voice, "My grandmother lost her leg and then she died. I don't think I can face this." The obvious thought being projected is: *It was a bad experience for her. Maybe I too will die next.*

On the other hand, some people have been exposed to a positive experience from an amputee. One logger had a large crane fall on his leg. He spoke in serious but confident tones as he stated, "My father lost his leg years ago in the war. It's been a nuisance for him but not bad. I'll be ok."

The present media has aided in the projection of positive

amputee role models. It seems popular to show individuals who have achieved in a variety of sports (skiing, track, basketball, soccer) in spite of limb loss. This visibility has encouraged many amputees, and others, to get back in the mainstream. They let themselves be more visible like wearing shorts and swim wear. Their confidence allows them to remove their prosthesis for some activities and try new things. A skier in a handicapped sports program was amused by all the attention. He said with a grin, "I was an amputee before it was fashionable!"

Most people have no personal connection with an amputee. Their thoughts of being in this 'club', as some have called it, can be confused and inaccurate. His thoughts as he lies in the hospital bed contemplating the future with a missing extremity may range all the way from the 'Bionic Man' to the beggar on the street. *Where do I fit in the picture? Will space age technology make me as good as (or better than) new? Or should I be stocking up on pencils to sell on the corner?* Most people with a new amputation have significant and understandable anxiety about their future life and function.

It is during this anxiety stage that a positive peer visitor can be truly helpful. The visitor is ideally another amputee that this person can relate to and who has moved forward successfully with his life. When I was recovering in the hospital my doctor arranged for a middle aged lady to visit me. She was a well-groomed school teacher who walked in smoothly in her dress and high heels. She shared her story of being thrown from her boyfriends' sports car years ago when a train hit them. It ran over her leg. The relationship didn't survive but she later married and had a good life. Later she drove me over to her home for another visit. She reassured me that driving a car without a stick shift was quite easy with her prosthesis on the gas pedal. Such encouragement was a treasure, even though many things about her life didn't fit mine. I was more athletic and outdoorsy and was growing in faith with all that was happening to me. This was not her approach but my vision of her recovery and return to a satisfying life was immeasurable.

The main factor to a successful peer visit is that the person with the new amputation is ready for it. In some of the early stages, meeting with an amputee is the *last* thing they want. They may be still struggling with the reality of it all. Always ask a person if they would like a peer visit before you attempt to arrange it.

3 ACCEPTANCE

For many people, their first area of concern relates to being accepted by others. *Will I still be loveable to the people closest to me? Will my spouse still choose to be with me? How is my family going to take this? Can they accept it? What about my friends?*

The answer to these questions lies in the fact that none of us had a perfect physical body pre-amputation. Even if we were attractive, it was not our external body that made us loveable. We are loveable sometimes just by being someone's child or close relative. A mother's love for her child is usually not affected by appearance. Sometimes her love may even intensify with the less beautiful child.

Most people, who truly care, like spouse, family, and friends, are not put off by a surface change like this. They may find it hard to come to the hospital or they may not know what to say. Like the person with the limb loss, they may need time to get used to the change. But if they cared before they care now even more.

Amputation can also serve as a serious test of a relationship. Perhaps a relationship was weak or had serious struggles within. Issues had not been dealt with in the past or communication was lacking. A marriage may dissolve under the pressure of this loss. This is more so if the person with the amputation is irritable, overusing drugs, or has become a self centered jerk.

However, many new amputees are amazed at the overflow of compassion and attention. Some of it comes from individuals they hardly know. As with many tragedies, it will often bring out the best in people. Flowers, cards and visits may come from unlikely sources. It happened to me and occasionally their acts of caring would bring me to tears.

Like me, another man confided, "I haven't really cried about this (amputation) but some unexpected people have shown they care. That makes me cry." It's a moving experience to feel love and caring from people one hardly knows or who are actual strangers!

Our Attitude

The amputee's attitude is crucial in facilitating the comfortable acceptance by others. By taking an active role in putting people around him at ease, the amputee will reap the benefits of close contact from others at a time when it's needed most. A willingness to talk about the loss as well as some light humor on the subject will convey an atmosphere of ease. The visitor should not be concerned that this person will be overly sensitive to an inadvertent comment like, "My new car cost me an arm and a leg," or "I thought he was going to talk my leg off."

Of course, if it's a difficult day for you, it's alright to let your visitor know. You could say something like, "I don't feel like talking about the accident right now but I appreciate your coming. Please come back again," is a good way to keep support connections open. This limb loss journey is too hard to do alone. We do best with other people's support at every level.

We've been considering the multiple emotional adjustments needed by the new amputee. Where does acceptance come in? It is sometimes difficult to determine the extent of acceptance which a person has about their loss. Many new patients have voiced the message like one man said, "I accepted this amputation immediately when it happened. I knew my arm was gone right then and there. I don't dwell on it. I just move on." In spite of their adamant statements, it is highly questionable that anyone can truly adjust so quickly.

True acceptance is a process which incorporates much more than just the head knowledge that a limb is gone. It involves an awareness of the impact this loss will have on every part of our life. Even the fact of the physical loss takes more than an instant to incorporate into our mind. Otherwise new amputees would not 'forget' that their leg is gone as they jump out of bed to run to the bathroom. Nor would limb deficient people continue to see themselves as intact in their dreams for months afterward (as they do and I did).

Our senses show us a fact: a portion of my body is no longer there. Our brain says *that part will not be growing back.* But that limb has been there for many years, and for most of us, it has served us well in a variety of ways. For a period of time (which varies from person to person) we will look down quickly upon awakening to affirm the truth of the loss. Most of us look down with the wish that this awful reality is indeed not true but merely a bad dream.

Acceptance comes down the road when we take this altered body image and say, "This is how I look now." We don't have to **like** that look but merely accept the fact of it like we do with other bodily features (freckles, large feet, tall, short, etc.)

The amputee with a prosthesis may ultimately have two mental views of his body. One is without the prosthesis (in bed, bathing or swimming) and the other is with the prosthesis. In my dreams I began to see myself utilizing the prosthesis because I wore it so much. For example, instead of running up a hill in the dream, I climb deliberately and carefully up it with the use of an artificial limb.

Positive acceptance comes when we stop comparing how things were to how things are or when we stop comparing ourselves to others. A former U.S. President, Theodore Roosevelt, stated years ago, "Comparison is the thief of joy." How profoundly true this is.

One angry gentleman spent years comparing what he could do before with his current situation. He did heavy physical labor at his job and enjoyed working in the yard at home. His leg amputation at the hip, along with progressively deteriorating circulation, forced him to leave his job and limited what he could do in the yard. He complained about the unfairness of it all to anyone who would listen. He was unhappy with the whole experience and not about to accept any of it. As far as I know, he never did.

I was even guilty of using my amputation as an excuse in the beginning. It was so handy to blame for lots of things. It was the reason I was late, did poorly on a test, or, best of all, why that cute guy asked my roommate out and not me. *If only I didn't have this wooden leg my life would be fine!* It can be good ammunition for a pity party.

The 'Super Amputee'

Some may disagree with my next statement but it is my opinion that often the 'super amputee' is someone who has not truly accepted his loss. The 'super amputee' is one who is engaged in physical activities that are difficult and uncomfortable for whole-bodied individuals and therefore more so for amputees. This may include extreme levels of skiing, triathlons, mountain climbing, etc.

It is not really the activity but the attitude about the situation. Does he need to achieve or win at this sport to be a worthwhile person? Is he trying to prove his value or worth as a person by what he does? Or is he just doing it because it's fun, he wants to do it, or he's just curious to see if he can do it? Maybe it's been a big part of his life for years and he really wants to get back into it if at all possible. That different attitude creates a different scenario.

One young man I read about lost both feet to frostbite while mountain climbing. Most people with two prosthetic lower legs would not see rock and mountain climbing as reasonable pastimes. This fellow, however, sees this activity as a part of his identity and what makes his life enjoyable. It's perfectly natural, in spite of it requiring significant effort, for him to go back to the mountains. Another amputee may be trying to prove to the world that he is as good as, or better than, anyone else by taking on this sport. Again, it's the underlying attitude.

Many amputees, especially younger ones, will attempt a variety of activities just to see how capable they really are. Once they know they can, indeed, do something then they deliberately decide if they really want to do it on a regular basis. The 'super amputee' is a person who *must* do it to prove his worth. The typical amputee will do it for the same reason as other folks; the activity is fun, accessible and affordable, and adds a positive dimension to his life.

Need to Prove Something

Please consider what I am really saying here. It is only natural for many of us to attempt to resume the work and play that made our lives worthwhile before amputation. It's healthy and normal to challenge ourselves with some new activities just to see if we can to it. The unhealthy part comes when we are led to do something because we don't feel secure in who we are. We become driven, if you will, to prove ourselves to the world. Our self-esteem has been assaulted and we must reestablish it with physical achievements that are otherwise meaningless to us. Of course, one doesn't need limb loss to feel driven to prove himself. Some people were in the process of trying to prove something when their limb loss occurred. For others, it's a lifelong struggle.

Once I had the privilege of meeting a remarkable man named Henry Viscardi, Jr. He taught me a lesson on the subject of acceptance. Mr. Viscardi was born with deformed legs which he described in his book[iv] as "gnarled stumps". These limbs were eventually fit with prostheses and allowed him to walk, but not without difficulty. He exerted great effort to walk without aids like canes or crutches. I met him in his seventh decade of life. When he got up to leave the room he reached for his crutches and said with a smile, "I guess I don't need to prove anything anymore."

To me, that is the ultimate requirement of acceptance. The battle to prove something (strength, capability, sexuality, etc.) is relinquished. Our self-esteem is no longer caught up in the need to show ourselves and others that we are worthy people by what we can do or how we look. When acceptance of our limb deficiency is NOT there we are saying, often subconsciously, *I am not a worthwhile person because there is a gap in my physical body.* When amputees have that belief, it requires a lot of effort to try and constantly prove their value as a human beings. In reality there is really nothing to prove. We already have intrinsic value in just being human.

Identity

It appears that most new amputees face the question of their worthiness in the beginning because their identity has been shaken. *Just how much of 'me' is caught up in possession of all four extremities? How much of my body can I lose and still be me?*

The more mature, secure person will work through this question. He will conclude logically, *I am still a valuable person because I possess many abilities and talents that are not dependent upon that absent extremity; This loss is just another challenge to overcome. It does not change who I am*; or, spiritually speaking, *No matter what happens to this body I am still a valuable person in the eyes of God.* Most of us take a little while to come to the above conclusions. Unfortunately, some whole-bodied people as well as some people with amputations never do. Normally we all have our days or moments of low confidence or doubt.

The goal is to have the pangs of the acceptance struggle become momentary over time. It eventually becomes just a twinge of sadness or emotional pain when we see a dancer or skater move with effortless agility. The long distance runner or mountain climber is viewed from a distance. Of course, with serious determination we may be able to accomplish the above activities. But the expense and effort will be significantly greater than for the whole-bodied person. We may choose to focus on the normal efforts of life instead. Raising a family, holding down a job, and comfortable recreation are typically more satisfying in the long run.

Clothing can be frustrating. Items like shorts, short skirts, or short sleeves may be exchanged for clothing that covers more of our differences. Strapless high heeled shoes may be bypassed for safer mobility. These changes are hard and some of us will make dramatic efforts before we make them. Personally, I had a special high-heeled leg made to walk down the aisle when I married. It was an expensive effort but was important to me at the time. It wasn't too long after that that I found some dressy lower-stacked heels to wear for special occasions. Acceptance requires reasonable tradeoffs as we move forward with what is really important and works for the long term in our lives.

Risky Behavior

Recently a gentleman who had just lost his leg due to complications of diabetes stated, "My family says this is the best thing to happen to me and I agree. I was living a risky lifestyle and not paying attention to the care of my body. If this hadn't happened I'd probably be dead by now."

Many other amputees have admitted that they were doing risky things at the time of their limb loss. If it had progressed further, they would surely be dead. With some, it relates to a disease process like the man above; ignoring symptoms, avoiding medical care, and generally behaving counterproductive to his health condition. This can also include over or under activity, poor eating habits, tobacco, and improper drug use.

Some people's risky behavior is more overt and results in traumatic amputations. It includes driving a vehicle under the influence, being reckless, or careless in any way. Often just being on a motorcycle in traffic is high risk, even if the driver is driving defensively. Any lack of good judgment or carelessness which results in an amputation provides one with a measure of guilt to overcome in his emotional recovery. "It's hard to think about the fact that it was my own stupidity that put me here," said one new amputee from his hospital bed.

Mental Health Issues

Other individuals are dealing with complex emotional problems or actual psychotic conditions. They have done things to harm or even try to kill themselves in their emotional pain. This includes the person who jumps from an overpass, drives into a tree, or shoots himself. Some of these individuals deal with conditions like clinical depression, paranoia, or other mental illness. These behaviors make life complex enough, and now limb loss must be dealt with as well!

It appears that a person's life becomes dramatically more complex if his mental health issues resulted in limb loss. Daily life was an intense challenge before the amputation. Many health care professionals, family, and friends, may legitimately wonder if this is the impact that will put this person over the edge, so to speak. Will even more bizarre behavior result, and perhaps suicide? Sometimes heroic limb salvage efforts are performed on unsalvageable limbs for this very reason.

One gentleman had crushed both legs when his van impacted a guard rail. The doctor shared with the staff, "Normally we would amputate these legs, but since he's schizophrenic, we don't think he could handle that so we're putting heroic efforts into saving them." A couple weeks later the legs became infected and during the course of treatment, the man nearly died. Amputations were performed below the knees and, surprisingly, he did very well with them. He focused on the tasks of physical therapy, prosthetic fitting, and walking. He seemed to thrive on the attention he received for his achievements and positive outlook. He learned to walk well on his prostheses without aides.

Over a period of years our health care team has seen a similar positive response to amputation by several who had significant mental health disturbances. Where their lives had been chaotic and lacking identity, they now seemed to focus on the efforts required of this rehabilitation project. Previously their life had often made no sense and people just called them crazy. Now they possessed a visible 'badge of disability'. If life doesn't come together now it can be blamed on this obvious limb loss and not the psychosis. After seeing several cases like this, one of our orthopedists concluded wryly, "Amputation can cure schizophrenia." Though simplistic, there is some experiential truth to this statement in that it provides a previously missing focus for their life.

The mentally unhealthy individual often becomes task oriented. In the midst of the many tasks to amputation recovery, they may not be overly concerned with the emotional impact of the loss. I inquired of one man who had jumped from an overpass if he had feelings about his own actions causing the loss. "Oh, no," he replied, matter-of-factly, "I never really think about it."

4 ADJUSTMENT

Home

For many individuals their *work* is living independently, caring for other family members and maintaining a home. Returning to our tasks of life are typical goals for most of us even before we can go back to earning an income.

Getting our body systems back to functioning is the first crucial step. They've been assaulted with surgery and a variety of medications along with the disease or trauma that led to the amputation. Everything from our lungs to our bowels may require extra effort as they seek to do their job automatically once again. Re-attaining mobility with wheels, crutches and a prosthesis can be a huge effort.

Normal hygiene is an early goal. Even in the hospital I remember being given the clearance for 'bathroom privileges'. Before that I was too sick and unstable to even get out of bed. I had never considered it a 'privilege' but now I was allowed to go to and use the bathroom on my own! Limb removal can force a person to start over again in so many ways.

The next steps are shampooing hair, taking a shower, and getting dressed. Every little thing has become a project. Just figuring out how to do these things safely is an effort. There's a lot of effort that goes into determining what to wear and how the clothes will fit our new body image. There are too many tedious decisions. We just want to get clean and get dressed and get going! Oh, well, at least trimming our toenails goes faster.

We also need to figure out how to feed ourselves, cook, and grow, or shop, for food. Early assistance from such professionals as physical & occupational therapists, social workers, nurses, and prosthetists (people who make prosthetic limbs) is needed. Adaptations to our home, as well as provision of mobility aids can make a tremendous difference. Do we need a wheelchair or crutches for a while? Perhaps, we need a ramp to get in the front door? Successful recovery includes attaining our previous independence, as much as possible.

Along with getting our body going, we typically have other responsibilities to return to. We may have a family and pets to care for. As a homemaker we may need to return to cooking, laundry, and caring for our spouse, children, and elderly relatives. The pets need feeding, grooming and exercise. Keeping the home clean and orderly and maintaining a yard are part of the job. Ultimately we hope to become an active member of our community.

Driving

In our and many other cultures the ability to drive is an important part of an independent lifestyle. It allows us to go shopping, travel with ease, and get to appointments. Distance walking and taking public transit with a missing leg or legs, takes much more effort. In the beginning, I was so grateful to be able to drive as I went back to school and work. One person with a recent amputation made the appropriate statement, "Take my legs but don't take my wheels."

Following my own accident, it became reasonable to transfer to a university nursing school near my home north of Seattle, Washington. Even with driving, I had to get to my different classes on a large university campus. Our body is trying to get used to the profound change of wearing a prosthesis as we attempt to further our education and/or get back to work. This effort can be immensely frustrating and difficult, but not impossible. In the end, achieving a certificate or degree of accomplishment can have so much more meaning. And getting that first paycheck is delightful. We are still valuable, productive people!

Work

For some people, their job is a primary concern following their amputation. This is especially so if they lost an extremity that seems crucial to their particular work; like the casino card dealer who lost his hand.

Multiple questions arise. *Can I go back to work? Is my job still available? Can I do it as well as before? What about safety and keeping up with my coworkers? Can I be a cost effective employee for my employer?*

As in other activities, the individual can often still do the tasks of their job. The real question is whether they can do these tasks quickly, efficiently and safely. Can it be done all day every day in order to earn a living? The new amputee should look at this carefully and realistically. There is no doubt that the carpenter with an amputated leg can build a deck on his house. But perhaps building houses is now not the best choice for his full time occupation. Some people make the wise shift to using their brain and experience more as in positions of quality control, management, or drafting.

Becoming a nurse was not a lifelong goal for me but it became one during the year of nursing education before my amputation. I did not consider that being on my feet for eight (or more) hours was not a good idea as an amputee, especially a new one. Fortunately, nursing, like other professions, has a variety of work areas. When hospital ward work became too demanding, I transferred into the nursery. Babies are easy to lift. The nurse may have periods of sitting when feeding or rocking them. Then I transferred to the night shift where transporting, lifting, and moving adult patients was less. With higher education, I was able to become a clinical nurse specialist in the care of those facing limb loss. Counseling, facilitating a support group, and networking for the patient's best health care all required less ambulation. Ultimately it became an ideal career fit for me. But it took time and a lot of effort.

One middle-aged lineman was determined that he wanted to continue in his profession where he had extensive experience and received great satisfaction. An electrical burn had cost him his forearm but with a durable prosthetic arm, he could, indeed, do the tasks of his job. This required support from his employer and determined effort on his part. He found the effort worthwhile as he reestablished himself in the work he enjoyed.

Some folks with a new amputation see that this is the opportunity to change vocations. It's not how they would have planned it, but now they can access the job training or return to school because they must. Before, they couldn't take the time off to pursue the job goal that was only a dream. An example is a logger who went back to school and became a draftsman. His above-the-knee amputation is no longer overly stressed by the demands of his new vocational choice.

More than one amputee has conveyed a real appreciation for this legitimate opportunity to change vocations. A mill laborer said, "I really didn't enjoy my job at the mill but it paid for the groceries and I sure couldn't take time off for school with the family and all. Now I can finish college like I always wanted and go for that engineering job."

Another said, "I knew I didn't want to stay with the heavy construction work forever. It gets harder as I get older. This is a good time to get that welding shop going that I've had in the back of my mind all these years." His tragic limb loss became his opportunity.

Play

Most of us have activities that really make our lives worthwhile. These are the fun things we do with friends and family and the refreshing and creative things we do alone. It includes playing ball with our kids or grandkids, golfing with friends, or fishing. Maybe it's the relaxing activities of card playing, gardening or painting. Or perhaps more aggressive activity, like snow skiing, hunting or playing team sports.

One of the first questions that the new amputee will typically ask is, "Will I be able to walk (run, jog, ski, swim, play basketball, play piano, garden, etc.)?" The obvious concern is that his life may have lost a big part of its value and enjoyment if his recreational activity is now gone with his extremity.

Fortunately, the reality for most amputees is that they can do many activities that they did before. The difference is that they often have to make some kind of adaptation in their performance of it. For example, the leg amputee can go hiking but usually not as far or as fast as before. And on uneven ground, a walking stick is an obvious advantage for balance. As one fellow with a leg amputation said, "I do what I did before; I just have to think about it first."

Skiing is accomplished with a wedge in the heel of the ski boot on the prosthetic side or the prosthesis is not worn at all. The ski poles may be substituted by 'outriggers' with small ski tips on the ends instead of the baskets and tips.

The arm amputee can utilize a variety of terminal devices (substitutes for a hand) on the prosthesis. This permits gardening, cooking, carpentry, or painting pictures with relative ease.

One of the more difficult challenges for the arm amputee is playing musical instruments. It can be more workable when the prosthetic arm is delegated to strumming or playing the chords. The electric keyboards also make limited dexterity easier. One gentleman with a below elbow amputation, told me that the only thing he really couldn't figure out was how to play the accordion.

Another man who lost both arms in a wood chipper injury, found much satisfaction in playing the harmonica. He was a happy fellow who, like the first, just wanted to make music.

One thing I have found as a clinician is to *never* tell an amputee that he will not be able to do something. This will either discourage him or he will strive to prove me wrong. The human mind is extremely innovative and can come up with a variety of ways in which to climb rocks, water ski, shoot a bow and arrow, golf, or play soccer – with or without extremities. It is best to let the person decide for themselves if they can or even want to do an activity.

The real limitation is when a person feels he needs to perform the activity in exactly the same way as he did before or 'it's just not right'. One fellow said he was rowing a boat with a special prosthetic ankle and another rower told him that he couldn't row that way, it wasn't 'right'. The amputee indicated that it was 'right' for him and verbalized rather forcefully that the two-legged rower should mind his own business.

The important thing is that we continue to benefit from the activity. That benefit may be physical, mental, spiritual, and/or social. Whatever makes it enjoyable makes it worthwhile. Fortunately, most people, unlike the two legged rower above, are supportive and share our excitement as recreational activities are resumed.

Camaraderie

Finding another person with a similar limb loss can be a huge advantage. When I found another person who skied with a prosthesis, it became much simpler. Among other things, he advised me to put a plastic bag over the prosthetic foot. This made it so much easier getting the boot on and off – and kept the foot dry besides! Like all of life, there are so many things to learn. Let's get help from each other and minimize the effort.

There is a loneliness in any crisis. A good visit with a person who has survived limb loss and moved on can minimize that alone feeling. It can provide a vision of hope when it seems like so much is lost.

Also, in a support group of people facing limb loss, we can

often find others that we can relate to and can learn from. Of course, there will be others in the group we may have absolutely nothing in common with except a missing limb. Every individual is so unique and so are people with missing limbs. We seek the ones who instill hope in us as we move forward with determination and purpose.

The support group is also a good place to establish camaraderie as we practice the humor in it all. Several of the members I've met shared humor in their own way.

One man said wryly, "I'm a foot shorter than I used to be."

Another said, "I became a member of this select group quite by accident."

And yet another joked, "It's hard in the shower when I try to jump up to wash the bottom of my foot."

A recovering alcoholic stated simply, "I admit, I drank my leg off."

An athletic young fellow stated about baseball, "I can still play the game. I just need to hit a home run to get to first base."

Internet

The internet is the way so many of us connect now. It is so easy! We don't have to transport ourselves to a group or an individual. We can connect through a variety of social media. One of my current favorites is an ongoing post on the website of the Amputee Coalition of America.[v] How I wish this would have been available when I joined this select group back in the 1960's. Like other connections, some of it doesn't fit me at all but the rest of it can be pure gold. The wall of aloneness is broken down and the 'amputee survival wheel' doesn't have to be reinvented over and over.

Legal Issues

As a final note to this adjustment process, I would like to briefly address legal issues. Our society is currently very focused on suing in an attempt to put a dollar value on people's losses. Realistically this cannot be done because there is no accurate value for a person's life or limb. It is often pursued anyway for a variety of reasons. Often it's motivated by the profound medical expenses involved. As one young man said, "It's not really the railroad's fault that I lost my legs but I don't have any money and someone's got to pay!"

Even if we, as the victim, are not inclined to sue, our friends and family may promote it. As one friend said, "Wow, you'll never have to work again! I'd sue them for all they have!"

A book could be written on this subject. The point I want to make is that legal recourse can have a negative impact on the person with a new amputation. Our court system is not speedy. As we wait for our case to be processed, sometimes several years, our rehabilitation can be significantly delayed. Sometimes the attorney actually advises that we not go back to our life of work, skiing, or other worthwhile activity just yet. The more pathetic we look when we arrive in the courtroom, the more money we (and the lawyer) are inclined to receive. This is just a fact.

We may lose, and losing a legal suit can be devastating. It becomes a second loss. Even winning can be disappointing. The win brings some money but our limb is still gone and we're not happy like we thought we would be. The money didn't fix our situation or our emotions.

Obviously some people need to utilize the legal system as they process their case, fairly. I want to encourage people to keep the big picture in mind if this is pursued. The goal is to get our life going again, not try to get rich. The two are not the same.

5 SAVING A LIMB

"The most important thing is to save his leg at all costs! Call in the experts! Money is no object!"

These were the anxious, commanding words of the distraught father. His young adult son had sustained an open (compound) ankle fracture from a fall while climbing in the local mountains. The wound had been grossly contaminated from the dirt and debris and already infection was setting in. The lower leg bones were shattered in multiple small pieces. Only one blood vessel, having been repaired, now provided the life giving blood to his left foot. The most irreparable injury was nerve damage. Though the foot was temporarily warm and pink, it was also numb.

Rapid administration of antibiotics soon controlled the infection. An outer framework of rods and screws called a 'fixator' held the bones together. The shattered bone pieces had been removed and now a three inch gap was left between the broken bones of the lower leg. Still only one blood vessel remained to feed his numb foot. The young man was strongly advised to consider amputation. The father was adamant that this was NOT an option and threatened to move him to another, 'better' hospital.

Parents

When a tragedy strikes our offspring, its effect seems magnified many times more than if it had happened to us. I have never met a parent who would not gladly take the place of their child in that hospital bed. It's immaterial whether the child is small or a full grown adult. Our child is always our child. To see him hurting and mutilated can be unbearable. Somehow as a parent we feel we should have protected him from this or at least now be able to relieve his suffering. But we feel so helpless.

Patient

When limb loss is a threat, tremendous emotions are stirred. The patient certainly does not want to say goodbye to a part of his body that is near and dear to him. When a person is threatened with loss, those close to him also experience the threat. The patient and the network of his significant others are now thrown into the crisis of this unwelcome situation.

Doctor

Even the doctor is highly reluctant to perform such drastic surgery. He/she went to medical school to save lives and fix people. Often the doctor's inclination is to take on the challenge and attempt to fix the limb even if the outcome appears bleak.

The important consideration here is not to let emotion do the deciding. The facts of the case must be weighed heavily. Can the limb be saved? Will the effort threaten the patients' life, quality of life, or more of his body?

Survival

The urgent need to remove a limb may come from spreading infection. The body becomes sicker as the invading bacteria travel through the bloodstream. If the source of the problem is not removed, the person will die along with the limb. This was my own situation after the boating accident. The doctor came soberly into my room around midday and said, "Dee your leg is infected. We have to take it off this afternoon or it will kill you. Do you have any questions?"

I shook my head, knowing that I would burst into tears if I said a word. So I waited until he left the room. Then I sobbed as the harsh reality settled into my heart and mind.

Body preservation

Although it seems highly illogical that a person would sacrifice their life for their limb, it infrequently happens. Cases I can recall typically involved feet that developed dry gangrene due to a lack of blood supply.

One homeless man adamantly refused the surgical removal of his dry blackened foot. He lived in and around a bus station in a small town near Seattle. Though he was a bit odd and inappropriate at times, he was rational, so the surgery could not be forced upon him. Once while a nurse was changing his bandage, a blackened toe broke off. Since the man refused treatment, he was soon discharged. He also refused offers of institutional care and went back to living homeless. We learned that he died a short while later due to ultimate infection in his system beginning with the dead foot.

Another woman was hospitalized in August with a darkened leg which lacked blood supply. It was soon amputated above the knee. The resulting wound was slow to heal due to her diseased vessels and her continued smoking. Just before Christmas, her other foot developed dry gangrene so amputation was again advised. She was a single woman in her mid-sixties who had determined that she did not want to live with both legs gone. The long hospital course seemed to have drained her energy and motivation. The effort of extensive rehabilitation and being wheelchair bound was beyond her. She died in March with her dead leg still attached. She was a weary but rational woman who chose a course that was difficult for us hospital staff members to understand. Over the years I have encountered a few others who would also, "rather die in one piece" than live with altered bodies.

But let's return to the more typical individuals who know that when life or limb is the issue, there is no question. The discussion goes something like, "Your arm has an aggressive infection. We must take it off today." or "The surgery did not open up the blood vessels enough. We need to remove the foot to above the ankle." When it gets to this point, most people don't argue.

Sometimes, in a case of multiple injuries, a person's chance of survival is enhanced when a questionably salvageable limb is removed early on. One fifty-six year old man sustained multiple, severe injuries when his motorcycle crashed. One ankle was crushed and nearly amputated at the scene. The other leg, and one arm, had bad breaks, along with his ribs. A week later the crushed ankle was determined not to be salvageable and was removed. He underwent multiple operations but after a few weeks he died. It appeared the massive injuries along with the extended hospital interventions, were too much. In retrospect there was some medical discussion that removing the crushed foot/ankle immediately *might* have helped save his life. His system could have then focused on healing the other injuries and not been further drained by a limb that appeared irreparably damaged from the beginning. This requires aggressive and early decision making on the part of the medical team and patient. It's a hard call.

Often in cases like the one above, the tissue from an amputated extremity is utilized in the other injured areas. For example, the bone, skin, blood vessels, etc., of this amputated limb are used as grafts for the other injuries. The phrase, "ultimate recycling", has been used in these situations.

In another case, a commercial fisherman sustained an open shattered fracture of the lower left leg. Attempts to save it made use of an outside metal framework. Following hospital discharge, the pin sites (places where the narrow rods of the metal frame enter the skin and bone) became infected. It moved up the leg and caused infection in the knee. Thus the effort to save the lower leg resulted in a higher amputation above the knee. Had the amputation been completed immediately, the knee could have been saved. Again, it is a very hard decision to make early on.

Saving The Unsaveable

Clinically speaking, an unsaveable limb is one which puts a persons' body or life at high risk. The above cases illustrate one of the most common errors in medicine today, which is saving a limb that is not save-able.[6] This error occurs for several reasons. Primarily, the patient is highly reluctant to part with his limb and the doctor is reluctant to remove it. Besides that, it is often very difficult to accurately predict, in the beginning, how it will turn out. Will the leg actually heal in the long run? And, if so, will it be functional and comfortable? If the person can't walk on it, what's the point of all the effort? Some of this is unknown in the beginning.

Among the more reluctant patients was the gang member who was brought in following a motorcycle collision. "If you cut my leg off, Doc, I'll have my friends kill ya," the biker announced. Even though the limb looked initially unsalvageable, the doctor did his best to piece it together in order to give the young man time to see the need for its removal. The leg was removed, *with the patient's permission*, a few days later.

Often a little time is needed for both the patient and medical staff to see the reality of the damage. If the patient did not see his injury initially it may be useful for him to view the wound at the hospital. For myself, I was amazed that my leg didn't drop off in the motorboat. So a later amputation was not a huge surprise.

Fortunately most reluctant patients aren't so threatening to the staff about the loss looming over them. They may refuse the surgery at first as they seek guidance and information from other doctors, family and friends. The average person will consider releasing a limb when the options and long term risks are carefully explained. Our body parts are near and dear. We don't let go of them without a struggle – nor should we.

Doctors' Struggle

As mentioned above, the doctor typically is inclined to attempt to save the limb if at all possible. It's their natural leaning. It feels better to fix a body than to remove its' parts. If accomplished successfully everyone is happier and other doctors are impressed.

Without significant experience (and sometimes even with it), it can be difficult to know in the beginning if a limb is truly unsalvageable. Early attempts are common to give the limb a chance and provide an opportunity for further evaluation. Unfortunately these early attempts to save often direct everyone's thoughts along the salvage mindset. It's often difficult to change that focus at a later date when much skilled time and effort on the part of the surgeon has gone into it. It can be agonizing for all involved to let go of the save-the- limb project.

Many people and some physicians truly believe, as one said, "It's better to have a bad leg than no leg at all."If you're dealing with a bad arm and not a leg, this statement may have some validity. However, with legs, in our society with quality prosthetics available, it often is not. Good lower limb prosthetic function for some people is sometimes not far below that of normal. Many people, including health care providers, are not aware of how quickly an artificial leg will surpass a damaged or deteriorating leg in comfort and function.

The thing to be especially alert to is 'ego' on the part of both patient and doctor. A person can envision themselves as a quitter or lacking determination if the salvage project is discontinued. Friends may say, "Hang in there. Don't give up." Too much attachment to the project can occur without thought to the reality of limited or no progress. Even the obvious deterioration of the person's overall health and his limb can be overlooked for a while.

Typically it is the doctor who presents the idea of amputation, as distasteful as the word may sound. Sometimes the patient is truly not aware that the long term outcome is looking as bleak as it is. Others feel they don't have the *right* to have their limb removed. "After all it's my body," said one woman, "I didn't think I had the right to remove part of it."

One gentleman experienced a severe arm injury in a car accident, with permanent damage to the nerves. His arm was totally numb. He kept the arm for over twenty years, receiving medical care frequently for serious cuts, burns, and scrapes to it. He was elated after its removal and described how 'free' he felt. When asked why he had not removed it sooner, he replied, "It was mine. I didn't think I was supposed to."

Ultimate Cost

The whole body is under intense assault when a limb is trying to be saved. High doses of antibiotics can produce kidney and liver damage, hearing loss, and other side effects. These drugs and their effectiveness for future ailments (strept throat, pneumonia, etc.) can be significantly compromised following the long term use needed for limb salvage.

People with diabetes and/or circulatory problems are often putting their general health and even their survival at risk. The extra required surgeries, being immobile, and in the hospital for extended periods can be outright dangerous. Getting rid of a dead or dying part, can often allow a person to get back a degree of quality in their life. Hard, aggressive decisions may be needed.

Parts of the body are sometimes donated to replace the damaged areas. Bone, skin, muscle, nerves, and blood vessels are often taken from healthy areas to fill in gaps in the damaged limb. These donor areas now have scars, sometimes pain, and may develop infections or limited function over time. One young man said angrily, following the unsuccessful effort to save his lower leg, "Now I not only have the amputation but I can't take my shirt off because of the ugly muscle graft scar on my back!"

The financial cost cannot be minimized. A dozen operations are not uncommon for limb salvage efforts. The associated hospitalizations and rehabilitation can easily amount to many times the cost of amputation recovery. This is true even when the amputation cost includes lifelong prosthetic replacement.

Long term function is being researched. Many health care providers, including this writer, have long felt that only a small percentage of salvaged lower limbs can outperform a modern prosthesis. Often a severely damaged limb that is saved requires an orthotic (outside brace) for support and protection.

A repaired limb which came close to amputation in the beginning will sometimes have a certain fragility and instability to it. Vigorous activities such as snow skiing, basketball, and soccer are among those sports that may be too risky to participate in. 'Normal' activities may be too much, such as extra walking, cycling, or a vigorous twist while golfing. A more sedate lifestyle may be forced on the person. Besides being less satisfying, this can have its' own risks over time (weight gain, blood clots, etc).

This unpredictability is especially annoying when it comes to employment. Being a reliable, capable employee who can keep up with the team is important to most of us and our employer. Missing work or being less attentive or capable on the job due to pain, etc., can make holding a job almost impossible. Even though prosthetic wear also has its physical irritations, they are often more predictable and manageable in nature. The user learns the degree of activity (how far and how fast) the prosthesis will allow and he can often be comfortably functional within those parameters.

In conclusion, the choice to remove a severely damaged limb is a hard one. The decision must not be approached quickly or without care. Many factors need to be considered. Ultimately it becomes an educated guess as to whether the original struggling limb will serve a person better than the replacements that are available to them.

An excellent editorial was written on this topic several years ago by internationally renowned foot surgeon, Sigvard T. Hansen, MD. It identifies the risk of saving a limb while ruining a life.[7]

6 REACTIONS OF FAMILY, FRIENDS, AND OTHERS

Two are better than one: For if they fall, the one will lift up his fellow but woe to him that is alone when he falleth; for he hath not another to help him up. Ecclesiastes 4:9-10

The sense of community is a crucial piece of our self-esteem. Indeed, how we are accepted and valued by others often determines how we see ourselves. It has been said that no one is meant to be a hermit. In our culture it's not usually demonstrated as the person alone living in the hills, but rather, the one who attempts to live with fierce independence within their community. Previous connections with family and friends have broken and new close ones are not established. There is often a subtle sense of pride at living independently. *I don't really need anyone,* is the inner statement of this self-sufficient person or it may be a more generous sounding statement like, *I don't like to bother others*. More often than not there is some pride that says, *I hate to ask for help – I can do it myself.* Some give this approach a vigorous try and even seem to succeed for a time…until a crisis occurs.

Getting through an amputation is not a crisis to be experienced alone. Connecting or reconnecting with the important people in our lives can make the project workable and will buffer the impact. We must be willing to make this connection.

When the reality of an amputation hits a person, one of their first thoughts is, *I wonder if this will matter to…(my spouse, fiancé, parents, friends, etc,).* Another thought is *,Who will ever want me like this?* Why does this occur? Why do we care what they think?

Several surveys have concluded that family support is an important factor to the successful adjustment to an amputation.[8] When it is not available, for whatever reason, the effort of coping can be too much. Just the tangible needs in the beginning are monumental. Help is needed for transportation to medical care, therapy, and prosthetic appointments. Home assistance for laundry, cleaning and shopping is also an early need.

As we apply ourselves to the hard work of recovery, our motivation may not be sufficient to just do it for ourselves. It is important to feel that someone else cares and that they are there for us.

They care that we are alive. They are happy when we smile, move and begin to re-establish our lives. They are our 'cheerleaders' who call, write, visit, and bring gifts. They will not be leaving now that there is something very different about our physical appearance. The burden of this loss is not just on our shoulders but they are choosing to share the load with us. This is empowering. We will recover because we have a life to live and also because we don't want to let these people down who have stepped out to help us.

Thankfully most of the people who really care will be there for us. They are like the young man's wife who lovingly told him, when his leg was crushed by a log, "You don't need ten toes for me to love you."

Often what has taken a part of our body also threatened to take our life as well. Our loved ones are grateful for our survival and usually willing to accept the revision of our appearance. Like us, however, they may need a little time to get used to the change.

Some won't be able to. I'll discuss that later.

Other People with Amputations

Connecting with other amputees is probably the most useful step a person with a fresh limb loss can take. It is an overwhelming feeling of loss for most of us when we first part with our body extremity. It reminds me of being lost in a forest with no clue on which way to go and how to get out. When we meet with another amputation survivor who has found their way out of the woods, we are given hope. Hope is the most powerful tool for perseverance.

Sometimes there are support groups nearby for people with amputations. Attending these can provide much useful information. We will not be able to identify with some people in the group but, chances are, there will be some who will be where we want to go. The group members are all at different stages of their own adjustment. Attending several times will expose us to the individuals and allow us to glean what is needed for our own progress. Some are doing well and some are not. It's important to meet both. As we move forward, it is also valuable for us to return to the group to help others.

The health care staff, often our prosthetist, may be able to connect us with a 'successful' amputee. The previously referred to national organization known as the Amputee Coalition of America keeps a listing of trained visitors that also have an amputation like ours. These people are available to provide a listening ear and understanding of the impact of what we are going through. Staff people tried to tell me that they knew of amputees who did this, that, and everything. But until I met one in person and asked a variety of questions, I was unable to grasp the hope that I desperately needed.

Others' Reactions

What about the people we don't know well? The casual friends, acquaintances, new people we meet and strangers. Their reaction is often affected by how conspicuous our limb loss is, as well as how comfortable we are about it.

Significant handicaps regarding our appearance are ones that are visible. It is hard to get past a severe facial disfigurement to get to know the person behind it. So it is with a limb loss. When it's our upper extremity or even a lower that does not allow for a normal looking or functioning prosthetic replacement, it serves as a barrier to people's early comfort and acceptance of us. They need to make a deliberate effort to get to know us. And some, for whatever reason, are afraid to do that or don't want to bother.

Personally, I like to give people the benefit of the doubt. Some will be startled at how I look with one leg. Frankly, if I saw someone like me at the public pool, I would take a second look too. There aren't that many of 'us' around. Most people have normal curiosity about it but don't know how to approach us. I guess it's more unusual for people not to take a second look. So if you *expect* people to look then you're fine when they do and surprised when they don't.

Humor

Remember to look for the humor in all of this. I don't think I can stress this enough. There is always something to smile about. Is it the startled guy in the shoe store who has grabbed your prosthetic ankle as he efficiently tries to slip on a new shoe? Is it the kid who innocently asks what happened to your *real* leg? It's best to laugh and roll with it all as you make yourself and others more comfortable with your revised body image. When we're too uptight or show our weariness of others' questions, we may inadvertently cut off the very encouragement and support we need.

I always work at making the airport experience as mellow as I can. That machine will beep in reaction to the parts in our limb. Expect it. The TSA people are just doing their job. Once a big burly fellow planted himself in front of me after the machine went off and LOUDLY asked, "ANY JEWELRY, BUCKLES, REPLACED JOINTS, CHANGE OR METAL ITEMS IN YOUR POCKETS?" I answered back, just as loudly, "ARTIFICIAL

LEG!" He dropped his voice and quietly called for a female agent. I smiled and stepped forward into the examining area.

Another comment that made me laugh came a couple of years after my amputation. When I married a young man who had lost the sight in one eye following the impact a frozen snowball when he was young; my ten-year-old brother asked innocently, "Will your kids have one leg and one eye?"

Negative Reactions

So far we've discussed caring, supportive family and others who mean well but may not know how to show it. What about those who 'can't handle this'? The ones who are extremely uncomfortable about the whole idea and would just as soon not be around you because of it?

Maybe it's your spouse. She married a buff young guy who was physically strong and able to provide support as an ironworker. Now he would be wise to choose another profession and will be challenged to maintain his fitness in the recovery and rehabilitation process. One ex NFL player said, "My wife married an athlete with 9 percent body fat and now she goes to bed with a fat, one-legged guy." That's a big change and not everyone is willing to make it work.

Most marriages and relationships have some struggles going on anyway. This amputation may put too much strain on an already troubled relationship. Sadly, it's a fact that some relationships won't survive this kind of impact. The good news is that, the ones that are strongly caring and committed will not only survive but be stronger than ever.

Sometimes the circumstances of the limb loss illustrate a problem in the relationship or with one of the individuals. Perhaps drinking or another drug abuse problem brought this on. Perhaps there was a refusal to let go of the nicotine use that was choking off the blood supply to their feet. Perhaps there was a refusal to seek medical care early on.

Risky behavior may have been a point of disagreement in

the past. Now your limb is gone and someone else was hurt or killed in the accident – maybe even your own child. Your spouse often said she didn't feel comfortable about whatever behavior was the issue. When the amputation is a visual reminder of a dysfunctional relationship, it can be too much and the relationship breaks.

Prejudice

Many people carry within themselves a prejudice against those with a handicap. They believe that for some reason those with a disability are less valuable or less human. Perhaps even a bit of a freak. They may feel pity for the disabled and, due to their own insecurities; they don't want to associate with these folks. *After all*, they think, *others may assume that they too are less valuable if they are seen in public with a disabled person.*

When something like an amputation hits close, like their family or close friend, a prejudiced person will either rethink or change their beliefs or they will completely separate from the handicapped individual. They may not visit at the hospital or later at home. As one fellow noted, "My card playing friends don't call or come over now. It hurts."

In the process of it all, a person with a new amputation may lose some friends or find that some people won't choose to be around them. It can certainly hurt or make us angry but when we really think it out; our experience can be an advantage. It's our own 'quality control' system. As one young woman said, "At first I was mad that he wouldn't ask me out just because I had an artificial leg. Later I decided he was actually doing me a favor because I didn't have to waste time on such a shallow man." This could most likely be the type of person who would leave a marriage relationship over a mastectomy or other disfigurement later on.

Dissupport

Not all people with this kind of prejudice will leave. What if it's your mother and you are her grown thirty-three-year-old son who has just lost his arm? She truly loves you but in her mind you have now become a useless cripple. Her grief is overwhelming as she wails, "My baby will never be able to take care of himself! He'll never find a wife! Who would have him?" So she steps in to take care of you and be the martyr mother covering everything from feeding to finances. When this kind of communication and negative interaction gets rolling it's called dissupport.

Dissupport can happen in varying degrees. Usually it begins as well intentioned and ultimately follows the premise that you are not and may never be the capable human that you could otherwise be if you had all your limbs. In contrast, positive support is available for what you really need at the moment. It's someone who is there and listens. It's a provider of transportation, cleaning, and shopping. Dissupport goes beyond. It often provides real support but to an extreme. It is the person who visits but insists on staying with you constantly without inquiring if that is what you want or need. This spouse, parent, child or significant other speaks for you from the emergency room onward throughout the rehabilitation process. Having an advocate isn't bad but this is above and beyond. She feeds, shaves, bathes, and coordinates every aspect of your care As you try to ponder the implications of your condition, you are tempted to think, *Well, I must be helpless now. She certainly thinks I am and I'm really not sure.* If you don't set your boundaries or get some distance from this person, you can easily end up being immobile, unemployed, and fully dependent. It is not a healthy place to be for anyone.

The ideal situation is where someone advocates for you and assists you *only as needed* in the early stages of recovery and beyond. Their very presence serves to assist in bringing you back to the highest degree of function in every area possible. It starts with letting you speak for your own needs and doing your own self-care, as you are able. It progresses forward to promote your mobility again and resuming driving, working, and playing. This positive person will not play the game for you but will be your cheerleader in getting you to do your best with what you have.

Supporters Need Support Too

The final area to consider in your personal support system is the fact that the people, who are trying to help you, may need help themselves. If they love you then they have also felt your loss. With a spouse especially, what you lose, she loses. She needs time to process it, grieve, and receive help from others also.

As one wife put it, "When I first saw his arm (amputated below the elbow) I was startled, repulsed. It took a little time for me to get used to it." Just as we need time to get used to our revised bodies, so do those that love us.

Small children may need a little more consideration but usually they do fine. One strong father had been injured in a construction accident. His two young children were coming to visit him and he was concerned how they might react to his missing leg. His wife was encouraged to talk to the children ahead of time about the injury, the hospital setting, and the missing limb. Typically the children are hesitant to approach daddy at first with so many strange things all around him. They may come to him on his good or intact side at first. They see that mommy is comfortable sitting next to daddy and holding his hand, and kissing him. It is not long, often just a few minutes, before the children are talking too, and comfortable with him. This is truly the daddy that they know and love, even if he is in a strange place with a missing part.

Impact on Family

The family is disrupted for a period. Siblings may feel ignored in the turmoil. My own sister told me years later, "I felt left out when you were getting all the attention. It was 'Dee this' and 'Dee that'. What about me? Am I still an important part of this family? I felt guilty for thinking it because I knew you needed help, but (at age thirteen) I still thought it."

Sometimes family can feel just exhausted from the effort of it all. They may be trying to keep the home in order along with a long distance commute to the hospital. The load can feel overwhelming, especially if other things aren't going well (car broke down, grandma's sick, dog died, etc.).

In view of all this, it is crucial that the family takes care of their own individual needs. Rest and good nutrition are crucial as well as brief distractions from the load like shopping, visiting, driving, walking, etc. There needs to be someone for the main support people to receive support from. The wife needs someone to talk to. If other family or friends are not appropriate or available to communicate with then professional counseling should be pursued. Often in the hospital there are psychologists or counselors available for the family as well as the patient.

A loved one's amputation is an unusual and highly stressful circumstance to be coped with. It is also one that requires recovery time. If a family uses all their energy in the beginning, it can feel like too much to carry out all the effort needed for ongoing medical care, therapy, and prosthetic fabrication later on. It's not a sprint, it's a marathon. They must pace themselves and incorporate any outside help that is available.

7 SPIRITUAL CONCERNS

Dealing with an amputation will challenge your belief system no matter what it is. You are out of control in this because you certainly preferred that you had not lost this limb. Since *you* are out of control, then Who or what is in control?

Is it just one of those things that happens in life? Is it fate or karma as some call it? If it is random fate, then why is my fate so devastating and other people seem to get off easier? Does it relate to bad choices I've made in my life? Am I being punished for wrongdoing?

Polls show that most people in our American culture believe in God[9]. From the standard Judeo-Christian view He is typically seen as an omnipotent Being who cares about us. In other words, He has full control over everything and has my ultimate well-being in mind. *If this is true then why didn't he stop this from happening? Is He displeased with me? I know I've done some wrong things but they don't seem deserving of this much punishment, if that's what this is. It seems that other people have done worse with no apparent consequences.*

Many people have reported that their faith has been crucial to their coping. They acknowledge that they have prayed. "Oh yes," said one burly mill worker whose foot was caught and crushed in a conveyor, "I've been praying alright, a lot!"

Other people don't seem to nurture their spiritual side as a part of their daily life and aren't about to start now. "No, I don't think about those things [spiritual beliefs]. I've always just figured things out for myself. Somehow I'll get through this," reported one motorcyclist with an above-the-knee amputation.

Personal Experience

A mixture of thoughts came to my own mind as I lay in a hospital bed after the surgery. I had made a decision to become a Christian when I was a nine-year-old child. Now, ten years later, I was struggling, grieving and afraid for my future. *Was my God still here and would He help me with this? Would that be sufficient for me?* Over the years, many of my patients have shared similar concerns with me.

One of my student nurse friends artistically painted in water color the Bible verse from Romans 8:28 for me. It states, "And we know that for those who love God all things work together for good, for those who are called according to His purpose." How I pondered the meaning of it as I read it over and over on the hospital wall in front of me.

"Well, Lord," I concluded, "It says you're going to make something good come out of this but I cannot understand how that can happen. Not from a tragedy of this magnitude. I'll just leave it up to You though, because it's too big for me to comprehend. Besides, I have some immediate survival projects to focus on." I needed to cope with the physical & emotional pain, make my body function and prepare for the next surgery. Theological questions were beyond me in the beginning, and sometimes still are.

I was able to comprehend some simpler concepts of my faith that also came from Bible verses. I knew that God loved me and He promised He would never leave me.[10] I was able to hang onto those truths and trust that, somehow, He and I were going to get through this. I had no idea how but I would leave that up to Him. That trust and His provision turned out to be crucial to my successful recovery.

Rather than feeling like I was being punished, I came to believe that God allowed me to go through this. Yes, He could have stopped it, but He chose not to. I was not a victim and I was more than a survivor. Most of my blood had to be replaced at the hospital. But I was kept from death for a purpose.

Another woman who lost her leg above the knee in a car accident shared a similar statement with me. "I know that this amputation was part of a Divine plan to grow my character and cause me to have more compassion for others," she confidently stated. These revelations don't often come early in the experience. This woman had lived with her amputation for over thirty years when she made this statement.

Other Faiths

One young man in my care was of Hindu faith. His hand was amputated at the wrist in a factory accident. His initial concern was a desire to continue playing a stringed instrument during their worship services. Since the missing hand was for strumming, it was determined that he probably could regain that skill with a prosthetic device, and he did.

A deeper dilemma was a part of this man's faith. He believed that this amputation was a part of permanent curse he would have to endure as he was reincarnated over time. That portion of his limb would always be missing, no matter what or who he became in future lives.

In contrast to this belief, the Christian anticipates a new, whole, healthy body in which to live out eternity. This hope gives us a different perspective. We only have to live with our amputation for whatever years are left on this earthly physical journey. I remember thinking clearly at age the age of nineteen that I may have as many as seventy years yet to live with this limb missing. That's not *forever*. I could do that.

Death

Most people who lose a limb have come very close to death. The accident could have easily killed us from the impact of the accident itself, bleeding or infection. For others the cancer, blood vessel disease or diabetes may still be, or feel, threatening. Life develops a sense of preciousness when there is an encounter with its end. Enjoying and appreciating each day at a higher level of purposeful living is often a very positive side effect of this amputation experience.

Some people don't take their close encounters with death in such a positive fashion. They may feel guilty that they survived and someone else in the same accident was killed. They may feel a sense of fear and futility in that a part of them has died with the amputation and the rest may not be far behind. Sometimes they may feel it would be better to be dead than to live like this.

Anger

It is not uncommon to feel anger towards God in this experience. *Why me? This isn't fair,* are common thoughts. A person's concept of who God is may become altered. If we thought *He is a 'God of love' but if He did this to me or at least allowed it to happen, then how does that fit? If he really has control but allowed this then He must not really care. Perhaps He is really a hateful being who zaps people at random, depending on His mood.*

Sometimes people develop an ongoing bitterness toward God or any higher power in their belief system. They think *I can't trust Him so I will refuse to have anything more to do with Him. Since He did this to me and I was not deserving of it, I will hold anger against Him and will never really trust Him again.* They stop attending services or following any previous religious practices, including praying.

It was not natural for me, personally, to be angry with God. I had been gifted with a loving earthly father. In spite of his obvious love, he caused me pain in some form when I lied or was disobedient. My dad once held me still while the doctor set a broken wrist bone. It was painful and I was afraid but I never doubted that my dad had my best interests in mind (although I wasn't so sure about the doctor). My dad had a purpose when he allowed or caused pain in my life. It was always for my ultimate well-being. My life experience has been the same with my heavenly Father. It's not usually obvious in the beginning but it has always been the best for me in the end.

Evaluation

It matters how your faith holds up in all of this. Maybe it's not sufficient. Maybe you need to explore what you really believe and who your god really is. Perhaps your belief system *is* sufficient but you have previously not really utilized it for your daily life or even for a crisis in the past.

You will get 'bitter or better' spiritually from this. Either you fight and turn away in anger or you thankfully trust a God who has your long term well-being in mind. So it has been with my Heavenly Father. I was hurting in many ways but I hung onto my faith. I knew I wasn't strong enough to get through this alone anyway. Ultimately even the Bible verse in Romans 8:28 made sense. God has worked this loss into a good thing for me and for others. I have been privileged to help many people in similar situations over the past fifty years.

8 BODY IMAGE & SEXUALITY

There is a picture in each of our minds of how we appear to others. We develop this sense through what we can see of ourselves and by using reflections, like a mirror or a photograph. We also utilize our other senses and communication from others to establish this vision.

This awareness is called our body image. It can be affected by simple things like getting our hair cut or colored. For some people just breaking a fingernail or having a 'bad hair day' can disrupt this image. Our body image can and does change with things like cosmetic surgery or permanent scarring from injury or disease. It certainly changes over time as we become adults, gain, or lose weight, and age.

My body image was blown out of the water, so to speak, when I started examining my swollen short leg with no foot. The swelling made it look like a club on the end, just below the right knee. Some of the hospital staff attempted to assure me that the swelling would eventually shrink dramatically. *How could I be sure?* This was all so new and scary. It just looked ugly and nowhere close to the lovely leg I had grown to appreciate as a teen. My tears came late at night when no one was around. How was I going to live with this, this stump of a leg? I hated it but could do nothing about it. So I prayed and focused on the work of therapy and learning to move safely again.

Our body image also impacts the way we move and how we function. We get sensory feedback from our body as we walk, eat, move and perform tasks. When we misjudge the presence of our body we can bump our shin, close the door on our finger or get the food on our face and not in our mouth. An athlete, dancer or entertainer is often extremely aware of his body's position in space as he performs after days and weeks of practice before an audience.

When there's a change in our body, we need time to incorporate it into our mind. One time, in the hospital, a staff member brought a stretcher in for me to scoot onto and go for wound treatment. I got up and took a step, totally forgetting that my leg was not there. She was on the other side of the stretcher and watched in horror as I went down. Fortunately, I grabbed for the stretcher and caught myself just as my 'short leg' was about to step into the floor. I only did that once.

Certain clothing alters our body image as it improves or diminishes our appearance or function. Consider a snowsuit, expensive formal wear, or a sweat suit. With a snowsuit we feel bulkier, walk more deliberately and may feel almost clumsy indoors as we reach across a table with fragile ceramics on it. The formal wear makes us feel and look more elegant and attractive. Women walk with more care in their high heels and enjoy the dainty beauty of the shoes. And, of course, in a fleece sweat suit we don't look our best but are usually delightfully comfortable and cozy.

Self-Esteem

Our body image can have a significant impact on our self-esteem. This is particularly so if being attractive to others had previously been easy to achieve and has become an important part of our identity. It can be threatening to lose a portion of that.

Some people who don't feel comfortable with their looks may try to enhance their appearance with clothing, jewelry, or a certain vehicle. We have all seen the air of confidence (arrogance?) exuded by the driver of a unique and expensive vehicle. To this person the right vehicle will provide, at least temporarily, a more appealing 'body image' or identity. One young man even made the statement, "When I'm in my truck, I look good."

It may go the other way for the person who cannot afford the nicer car or for some reason makes use of an older, well-worn model. A person may feel a sense of embarrassment or some insecurity at being seen in such a shabby auto. A bumper sticker I saw illustrated this in stating, 'You have to be really secure to be seen in this car'.

For most of us our attractiveness or lack thereof is one of the many features of who we are. Some people, however, have a large part of their identity, and sometimes their vocation, involved in their appearance. The beautiful or handsome model or actor is the classic example. One young man I worked with lost half of his hand in a fall. He was unconscious and lay on top of his hand for many hours, thus impairing the circulation. The disfigurement that resulted was devastating to him. "This ruins my life," he stated, "I am a model and a waiter. How can I present a plate of food to anyone with a hand like this?"

Coincidentally, I encountered another young man a few months later with a very similar hand injury from a sawmill accident. I asked him how he was doing emotionally with his injury and clarified that I knew some people would be quite upset. He shrugged and smiled, "Well, where I come from [a small logging town in Washington State], nearly everyone has something missing. I guess I'll just be like everyone else!"

One of my own great uncles was quite prosperous in the Oregon lumber industry and lost several fingers off his right hand in a mill accident. "A hazard of working your way up the lumber ladder," he stated wryly.[11]

After our adolescent years most of us don't have a strong need to look perfect because we begin to realize we really never really were. However, we don't want to look too different or mutilated either. We certainly don't want our appearance to cause adults to be shocked or children to cry. Understandably, we want to blend in and look as normal as possible, whatever 'normal' is. Typically that includes having all four extremities with ten fingers and toes.

A current song by R&B artist, John Legend, alludes to the depth of real love. The song, entitled "All of Me", not only overlooks imperfections in his loved one but sees them as part of her unique desirability. In his mind she is still perfect inside and out.[12]

Feelings about Sexuality

We were made from the beginning to be sexual beings. When part of our anatomy is altered, especially a part that we identify closely with our sexuality, our identity is threatened.

For example, legs are often viewed as a part of a woman's sexual attraction. And a man may see his biceps and broad shoulders as a part of his physical appeal to women. If a person loses one or more of these limbs, do they become less female or male? When an amputation occurs, that concern may become paramount.

For me, one of my first thoughts as I lay in the hospital bed was, *Will guys even want to date me with something like this (a missing leg)?* In the past I had received compliments on them and I felt that my legs were one of my better features. It was distressing to think about being less desirable and gave me a sense of uncertainty about my future. I hadn't dwelt on the idea too much but had always felt that I would someday get married and have a family. Now I wondered...

Several men have shared with me that just the mutilation of their body, whether it was a missing foot, leg or hand, made them feel 'castrated'. It surprised me how readily that term was used by them to describe the threat they felt to their maleness. A missing limb typically has little, if any effect on one's ability to perform the act of intercourse. It was obviously more than that. It was apparently the idea of being considered unappealing, or worse, because of the changed body. No one wants to consider that they may be viewed as repulsive at an intimate level. If someone is to reject us, we prefer it at a different level than our sexuality.

One lady met with me a few months after her amputation and expressed concerns about a possible suitor. "We've been friends for some time and he wants to date me. I can't imagine that he could find me attractive with this missing leg. What should I do?"

My advice to her was, "If he thought the idea of your missing leg was unappealing, he obviously wouldn't even ask you out. It's not a secret. He can see it's gone. Yet he wants to spend time with you anyway. Go for it."

Sometimes it's our own prejudices or presuppositions that enter into it. If we previously (or presently) would not want to be around someone with an amputation, then it's easy to assume that others would not want to be around us, especially at a sexual level.

Our attitude is crucial in all this. If I truly feel like less of a person because my body is altered, it is difficult for others to get around that and not feel the same way. As one fellow whom I later dated said, "Well it doesn't seem to bother you so why should it bother me."

However, there are people who will not date a person who has an amputation. That can be annoying and even provoke anger on our part. But when seen in perspective, that we aren't wasting time on a person with such a shallow outlook, it's to our advantage. That is the kind of person that you could marry and might later head out the door if you lost your hair or needed a mastectomy.

One young couple I met was extremely attractive. She was a model and he was a professional athlete. They had only been married a couple years when he lost his leg due to a serious injury in his sport. He put forth great effort to look and dress so his prosthesis wouldn't show. He maintained his physical fitness but felt he was unable to perform at the high level of athletic competition he once knew so he gave up his beloved sport completely. Unfortunately, his wife was unable to be comfortable with him on several levels, including physical intimacy. She avoided their previous enjoyment of showering together and required that he cover his shortened leg when they had sexual relations. For her own reasons, she had married a physically intact, handsome athlete. When he could no longer fit that image, she could not accept it. Sadly, the marriage did not survive.

Fortunately, most people are not so focused on physical perfection. Maybe it's because we all have some imperfect features, even before we dealt with any major surgery. More likely it's because, as humans, we have a variety of characteristics that make us attractive to another. Some of those characteristics have nothing to do with our appearance (sense of humor, faith, humility, intellect, etc.). Even our physical body has much more to it than one or two extremities. As one young husband commented regarding his wife's amputation, "Well, it's not the prettiest part of her but it comes with the package."

One middle aged couple seemed especially well connected. The husband had experienced a recent amputation while working at his long term job on the railroad. The wife was very attentive and caring without being demeaning. I mentioned it and she said with a smile, "Two years ago I had a hysterectomy and he took good care of me. Now it's my turn to help him get through this."

In the beginning, people are often concerned about their actual ability to perform sexually from the physical standpoint. Depending on the extent of injury and stage of recovery, creative people can find comfortable positions for intercourse. One young man asked me if it would even be possible. I inquired about his injury, which he described as a lower leg amputation and denied any groin injury. "Then there should be no problem," I concluded.

He later confirmed that I was right.

Of course, if you feel that you are actually unappealing to your spouse because of your body appearance, then you may limit your own ability to be responsive. That ability alone has many psycho-emotional factors involved. As one single man stated, "I couldn't imagine any woman actually wanting to go to bed with me." His own feelings then become a barrier to even initiating a relationship.

Some of us women don't appreciate that our 'presentation' is impaired by a missing leg. How does one slink into the bedroom with a new negligee either hopping on one foot, using crutches, or prosthesis? Even the best looking prosthesis is a bit clunky and provides a limp when 'barefoot'. And how do you seductively slip it off as you get into bed with your spouse?

One young man shared this story with his doctor. He had recently recovered from an above-the-knee amputation following a logging injury. He was a very handsome fellow and previously had no problem picking up women. He had gone to a bar with friends one night, wearing his prosthesis but dressed so it didn't show. He struck up an acquaintance with a young woman who eventually agreed to leave with him, but first he got up to go to the restroom. As he walked away she noticed his limp and asked his friends about it. They mentioned his injury and how well he was doing. When he returned to the bar the young woman was gone. The message seems to be that missing limbs (and probably most other disabilities) don't go well with what is loosely called, 'one night stands'. A relationship should to be established before sexual intimacy is pursued. This is not such a bad idea for folks without amputations either.

Devotees

This chapter wouldn't be complete without mention of a phenomenon where a person is specifically attracted to another *because* of their amputation. Some call it a fetish and some call it a legitimate attraction like to certain hair color or other body features. Typically this is an attraction that a male has towards a female with an amputation. There is a significant sexual arousal that accompanies it.

Many females are frightened and/or insulted that someone would pursue them only because of a missing limb. Yet I've heard other women indicate that they don't mind having their amputation draw in some men since it seems to repel a few others.

My personal impression is that, like most fetishes, it focuses too much on the body feature and not on the person. A healthy relationship is based on a wide range of aspects of one's personhood. The implication is that if, by science or a miracle, she could one day grow back the missing limb and she would no longer be desirable to this person. Quality relationships should go deeper than that.

9 SOCIO – CULTURAL IMPLICATIONS

What does an amputation mean in your society or culture? Does it imply shame, a curse, ugliness or uselessness? Perhaps it identifies you as a thief who was punished with an amputation? In some cultures during wartime, it may identify you as a victim or, perhaps, even a hero; one who fought courageously, giving up a part of your body for your country.

Our societies' view of an amputation cannot help but affect our identity and our own view as we ponder its' meaning. There are a wide range of biases by people in different countries and by social groups within those countries. Below are a few of the typical ones.

Pity

It is common and even understandable that an amputation may incur a feeling of pity by some people. As a very visible handicap, it shows that a person's body has less to it than other people.

Even though there is sometimes a sense of compassion and concern with pity, it has the downside of seeing the person as a lesser human. Many amputees have conveyed to me what one man said, "I can't stand it when they look at me with pity." It may simply mean, *I'm sorry that you have to live with an added challenge.* At its worst, the look of pity implies that *it's too bad that you have this unfortunate condition that will keep you from ever being what the rest of us are or what you could have been.*

Shame

Sometimes just our appearance can provide us with a sense that we are not as attractive or 'whole' as we would like to be. In times past, people with obvious differences would stay away from public view just because of this. Our unique appearance would have caused our family to keep us home and/or put us in a special school or institution for the disabled. Many societies continue to do this.

Even today, there are some who feel a sense of shame about their incomplete appearance, especially in the presence of others. This is in spite of great progress in some places to provide similar opportunities to all people. It is more prevalent in some cultures, families and individuals.

If we were completely honest, all of us who have limb loss would probably recall a time or two during our recovery when we felt a sense of shame about our revised body. It's often the reason that, on occasion, we have avoided public swimming, revealing clothing, or physical intimacy.

Uselessness

It is common, especially in the beginning, to wonder if we will ever be a productive member of society again.

People who have come from physically oriented jobs are particularly concerned as they consider that earning a living might be difficult if not impossible in their past vocation. This might include ironworkers, builders or roofers. The government may have a program that provides a disability pension which can be tempting to the person with an amputation. For some it is needed, but for others, with a clear mind and several remaining extremities, it is not. For those of us in this category, it is not to our benefit for the government to say or imply, "You just sit here and we'll send you a check to live on because we don't think you can do anything now."

This unnecessary rejection can also be reinforced by a military system that refuses to take people with even minor handicaps. As a student nurse I recall going with other student friends to the enlistment office during the Viet Nam war. I was not surprised but felt irritated that some policy makers saw me unqualified to serve my country just because of a leg amputation. It's unfortunate that many of the non-physically oriented military positions (clerical, music, driving, writing, etc.) are not considered at enlistment time as possible options for the handicapped.

Those who live in countries with less industrialization and more reliance on physical labor can feel especially threatened. It's not unusual to have an unemployment rate of over fifty percent in some of these developing countries. People with any limitations are at a great disadvantage in the competition for jobs. For these people the potential for becoming an instant beggar can be very real. A beggar is perhaps the epitome of feeling useless. Yet, in some places, being a beggar with the visible handicap of a missing limb can be profitable. In contrast to a low paying, or no job, it becomes a serious temptation.

Criminal

There are some countries and cultures that have for centuries, used amputation as punishment for a crime. If you are caught as a thief, your hand may be amputated. These cultures typically have a tradition of using their right hand for eating. Utensils are not common so people eat with their fingers. The other hand is used for dirtier jobs like toileting. To magnify the impact of the punishment, the right hand is removed, thus requiring the thief to eat with the 'unclean' hand.

Cursed

Religious dogma and ancient superstition can cause great fear and rejection. The person and their society may truly believe that their altered body displays the results of a curse. The intensity of it can cause parents to harm or kill their offspring in an attempt to minimize the curse on the rest of the family. In West Africa I have known of people leaving their handicapped baby in the jungle, starving them or throwing them in the river. Lest we think that in the United States we are morally above that. We are not. We merely act more sophisticated about it. We use medical equipment and procedures to identify a handicapped child *before* birth. It allows us to destroy them without ever holding them. In both cases an attempt is made to remove the curse and inconvenience of a child who seems less than whole.

This idea of being cursed is profound in some cultures. The family member with a limb loss may represent more than just showing that the person or family has been cursed. It may further mean that the person is an actual devil. One mother was told not to nurse her imperfect baby because the demonic powers would be transferred directly to her own body. She chose to let the baby starve than risk the possibility of that happening.

If a mother or other family member chooses to care for her handicapped offspring, she may face many social barriers. The father may leave his entire family in his need to not be associated with a cursed child. Any and all problems (infertility, weather changes, and money limitations) may regularly be blamed on the child. The extended family and community may verbalize constant rejection.

Even when demonic concerns are not prevalent, there can be personal thoughts of fear and guilt regarding a handicap. Parents may recall drug use or promiscuity around the time of conception. *Did my actions cause this in myself or my child? Am I being punished for my actions?*

Marriageability

I still remember the loudly-grieving mother at the hospital. Her beautiful teenage daughter had lost her fifth finger to an injury. To this Asian mother, her daughter was no longer perfect and therefore not marriageable. It was a tremendous loss to the family and to the girl.

When I travelled to El Salvador after their civil war, in the late 1980's, I commented that the many young soldiers with land mine amputations could probably find wives since it was such a common injury. A kind man corrected my thinking. He said that even if a young woman wants to marry a man with an amputation, she will be discouraged by her family. El Salvador is a labor-intensive culture and families looked for someone who could support their daughter and future grandchildren. A man with an amputation would be at a great disadvantage for such a task.

Women in a developing country face the same barrier. As a wife and mother in the prevalent working class, she will be required to raise and harvest crops by hand; carry wood, children and food;, wash clothes in the river, etc. These are monumental tasks for a young able bodied woman. The workload can be impossible with a missing limb; especially when prosthetic substitutes are limited or not available at all.

Changing Biases

Change to these attitudes is normally slow in any culture. Provision of mobility aides and prosthetics is a good start. Affirmative action by the government can be another great step in turning a person with an amputation from a tax user to a tax payer. In my own state, I was able to access school funding through the Division of Vocational Rehabilitation to complete my nursing education at the university level. Even with this assistance, I worked part time at a government affiliated hospital. It was to my advantage that they were required to employ some people with disabilities. Ultimately it was to my country's advantage that I was employed there for thirty-four years and became a lifetime taxpayer. What a privilege for me to be a productive citizen.

The media can also have a tremendous impact on changing biases. By making functioning, successful amputees more visible, people's mindsets can begin to change. Human interest stories about us working, running and playing show us not only blending into society but being productive members. This is powerful.

Stories about individuals who overcome in spite of the odds

are always inspiring. More developed countries have utilized this method for some time and many people with old biases have been forced to change. It's hard to see an amputee as pathetic, helpless and cursed when he holds a professional job and plays on a soccer team.

Our Part

Ultimately it is we amputees who have the power to change the mindset of others and, the culture we live in. This does not require heroism but it will take determination and tenacious perseverance. Everything truly takes more effort, energy and time, than it used to. We can work up a sweat as we strap on a prosthesis, walk across the room, take a shower and perform all the tasks of daily function. Sometimes it's not comfortable. It was often physically difficult for me to get across a large university campus for the classes needed for my degree. When our body has other issues like poor circulation or diabetes, it becomes profoundly difficult. We move forward because doing what we can feels better than not, and it *is* better.

When my own leg was removed during my first year of nursing school, I was determined to move ahead with my nursing plans. Some people saw this as heroic and even put my picture on the front page of the local paper with the headlines, "Student nurse who lost leg plans to continue with nursing!" This was a bit amusing and puzzling to me. *What else was I to do?* I knew that I liked nursing. *Do I now just sit down and cry in a corner for the rest of my life?*

Life still awaits us. For some reason we are still here. A life with a missing limb hadn't been in our plans. But it is still life. So we move forward the best we can. In the process people with less visible struggles are inspired. Some of them are encouraged by us as their biases fall away and they continue forward with their own less-than-perfect life.

10 FEELINGS ABOUT PAIN

Pain is a life experience. Having a body part removed is like all surgery – painful. It will happen either before, during or after the amputation, or all of the above. The focus here is, ultimately, how does the amputee feel about that pain, especially afterwards. Chances are; some of those feelings are quite normal.

Duration

When people think about pain from an amputation, some are concerned that it may be life- long. The alteration of the limb is permanent. An early concern is that perhaps the pain is permanent also. Once while working as a staff nurse, a hospitalized patient learned of my amputation and asked me what drug I took for pain. It had been fifteen years since my surgery. I told her that I took nothing. Her amputation had been a year ago yet she focused intently on it. She told me that since the surgery she had never quit taking pain medication.

Degrees of Pain

As mentioned above, pain is normal when an amputation occurs. Degrees of it will vary with individuals. First there is the initial pain that leads to an amputation. It may be a crushing trauma or severe blood vessel disease. Both of these can give a sense of the pain being unbearable. Common early feelings include, *I can't stand this pain. I'm going to pass out* or *I hope I pass out or just die. This is too much!* The amputation itself can be seen as a degree of hoped for relief from such an experience.

Of course, there are other pre-amputation conditions that are not too painful. Some people have limited sensation due to the nerve damage of their diabetes. Others have reported only minimal discomfort from a bone tumor. Still others have a chronic type of pain from an injury years ago. This can vary from intense and keeping them awake at night to being painful only when they walk or move too much.

The intense level of pain either before or immediately after an amputation can give one a whole new view of the pain experience. When '0' is comfortable and '10' is the worst pain imaginable, then the experiences of our pain fit somewhere in between. The mild toothache or headache, a two – three pain level; stubbing our toe or hitting our thumb with a hammer, a six – seven pain level; having a baby, a seven – nine pain level, can all fit a pattern or scale in your mind. It puts your pain experience in perspective. In many ways the lower levels of pain can now seem more tolerable *because they are*, in comparison.

Pain after surgery is, of course, very individual. It usually depends a lot on the persons' pain tolerance. Some of us can get shot by a gun and not know it while others will have a hangnail and the world will know it.

Drug Dependence

One factor that influences pain tolerance is past drug use, legitimate or otherwise. The use of pain medication for an extended period causes our body to become accustomed to drugs of this type. Now when the pain increases from surgery, the normal dose of medication will not be as effective.

For myself, I have always tried to avoid all pain medicine except when absolutely necessary. Having experienced unbearable pain when the boat propeller hit, I am eager for my pain medication to work hard and fast should I ever need it again.

Illegal or recreational drug use is a magnified problem.

People who indulge in this behavior consistently will typically have very little tolerance for pain. Everyday life is usually 'a pain' to them, which is why they often take the drugs in the first place. Sometimes, as a result of reckless behavior while under the influence of these drugs, real physical pain occurs. Then they often have limited ability to cope with this pain either physically or mentally. They sometimes will overreact with great complaint to common exam procedures like blood pressure measurement, or needle sticks. As a nurse in a Trauma Center, I observed regularly that long term drug dependence (alcohol, marijuana, prescription meds, etc.) can make pain very difficult, if not impossible, to manage.

Pain Following Surgery

Of course, the interventions of the surgical team can make a big difference at the time of the amputation. Some people get a significant level of pain relief from an epidural or spinal type anesthetic while others do well with certain narcotics. These people will report absolutely no pain with the above interventions. Conversely, there are a few that will report no relief from their pain with anything. Most will have a post-operative pain experience somewhere in between.

The interior of bones are loaded with nerves. The pain is intense when they are broken, intentionally or otherwise. This pain is a safety feature that keeps us from moving our limbs or walking on them and allows them time to heal.

Commonly, all bone surgery, including amputation, results in high levels of pain for two to three days. Often there is a significant drop in pain after that period, as long as the revised bone is kept protected and moved carefully. It goes from serious pain to discomfort that is later described as soreness, tenderness or achiness. Initially strong drugs are needed but after a few days the revised limb discomfort is managed with non-prescriptive pills, change of position and focusing on something else.

Becoming a Survivor

An early positive part of this experience is that a person may become aware that he has now survived a significantly traumatic experience. In many cases an amputation has occurred from a close encounter with death itself. Often the surgery was performed to avoid death from a tumor, infection or lack of blood circulation.

It can be empowering to grasp that we are still alive when we came very close to not being so. This empowerment can cause us to work with and take charge of our pain. This is especially so if and when we realize that the worst pain is now behind us.

People don't always grasp this 'survivor' title and those that don't, often see themselves in the role of the 'victim'. Being a victim for a short while is not necessarily bad. It can help in claiming the truth of the loss and expressing normal grief. However, if we don't move past being a victim, our life will have an added emotional burden. This is especially so when we see the amputation as the death of a part of us and consider that perhaps the death of the rest of us is not far behind. Or we may keep comparing ourselves to how our intact body used to be and hang on to grieving for too long. Perhaps more frustrating is the comparison of how others' bodies appear whole and fully functional and the accompanying sense of jealousy.

The healthy approach is to become a survivor; grateful to be alive and eager to see what life has yet in store for us. A survivor can then become an overcomer. We come to realize that future challenges of life can also be successfully faced and overcome.

In summary, pain is merely an alarm system. It can become dysfunctional but we should see it like a smoke alarm. It should only be turned off temporarily as the cause of the smoke is dealt with. We don't remove the batteries and leave them out. It's the same with pain. We don't take drugs constantly or keep cutting off more of our limb just to deal with our discomfort. We deal with the problem as best we can and then move on with life. It becomes our choice whether this pain is abnormally focused on. In all of life, "pain is inevitable– misery is optional".[13]

11 PHANTOM FEELING

There is a sensation that most people have with an amputation experience which is called the 'phantom feeling'. It sounds kind of spooky but it essentially is just the feeling that the amputated part is still there. It's relation to body image is that our senses are now giving us a different message than reality. The individual sees that his foot is gone but can still feel it. It's similar to the feeling we have when removing our hat and yet it feels like it's still on. Or taking off a watch to get in the shower and yet the watch feels like it is still there.

Words are powerful. For this reason I choose to use the term phantom 'feeling' rather than phantom 'pain'. This feeling is not necessarily painful and we don't want to assume that it will be. However, if we call it pain, we are more inclined to struggle with it rather than just accept this odd sensation and move on. This is not to say that we may not have significant discomfort from it at times. But usually it is fleeting, especially when we can distract ourselves with activities of life.

If a person goes into an amputation without knowing about the probability of phantom feeling, he may become frightened by it. One woman was stunned to feel her missing foot after the surgery. She told me, "I knew I had lost my leg and now I thought I was losing my mind!"

What exactly is phantom feeling or sensation? Essentially it is the sense that the missing extremity is still there after it has been physically removed. Neurologists describe our brain developing a type of 'nerve map' of our entire body before we are born. Later, when a part is removed the brain's map is still intact. It's not unlike the camera card being removed from the computer. The pictures still are visible since they were stored in the main computer memory (or RAM). The brain's map is beginning to get different nerve feedback from the missing limb. The limb stays in its memory but becomes somewhat jumbled with these new sensations. The limb feels like it's still there but often feels very different and these feelings can change over time.

Although most amputees feel something, there are a very few who report never having phantom feeling of any kind. These reports appear to be specifically from people who had numbness in their extremity before the amputation. This numbness is typically caused by nerve deterioration, like in diabetes. In some cases it can be brought on by medical intervention where the area is intentionally made numb a few days before surgery.

Phantom sensation can be highly annoying. Some people call it different names like 'ghost pains' or 'electrical feeling'. One man referred to the tingling in his missing foot as the 'flight of the bumble bees' and another said they were like 'sparkles'. It typically feels like the part is still there but sort of like it has fallen asleep and tingles. At first it can feel very different and fairly intense with the fresh injury to the nerves. As it heals, the feeling diminishes for most people and they become accustomed to it as well.

Sometimes it may be described as 'an electrical jolt', similar to the feeling of hitting your 'funny bone' [nerve at the elbow]. Other descriptions are stabbing, burning, cramping, twisting and aching. Fortunately, for most people, the intense phantom feelings are short lived and sporadic. However, these feelings are typically more prevalent after surgery or with an open wound in the area. This is due to the irritation and exposure of nerves. Fatigue will also magnify the phantom. Leg amputees, including myself, have often found this after a long hike. An arm amputee may experience it after much repetitive motion.

Like all pain, the phantom discomfort is magnified by attention. The more we think about it or focus on it, the worse it gets. One strong, young logger experienced a leg amputation when a tree fell on him. He was recovering well and after a few years came to the clinic for a new prosthesis prescription. While there he volunteered to answer questions about phantom pain for a study being done. He reported, after completing the form, "I never had phantom pain before but I do now."

Phantom

The phenomenon is still not fully understood but has to do with the central nervous system being disrupted and not knowing how to adapt to the change. On the other hand (pun intended), a person with a hand or arm amputation will often have a very strong sense of the missing hand. Often they can describe a ring or watch still in place. This sensation is believed to be stronger in the upper extremity because of the prevalence of nerves for touch in the hands and fingers.

The phantom feeling thrives on attention. After 50 years I can still feel my foot and even wiggle my toes. But I'm usually not aware of it because I'm so used to it. It's not a bad feeling but it feels different than my real foot. I try to describe it like the loud sound of the river that campers hear as they are setting up camp. At first it is very noticeable, almost too loud. But as they get settled in, they hardly even notice it.

One young man came in for his early clinic checkup regarding his below-the-knee amputation. "These phantom feelings are very annoying. When will they go away?" he complained. Three months later he returned for his routine clinic visit. He had a young family, had returned to his office job and was getting back to playing golf. We asked how his phantom feelings were. "Oh, they're still there but I don't pay attention to them anymore. I'm too busy."

Some people are afraid to admit to their phantom feeling. It hasn't helped that some psychological literature has suggested that the feeling is not real or that it has a psychosomatic ['all in your head'] aspect to it. A few professionals have even suggested that there is some wishful thinking going on. The idea is that we who have missing limbs would like them back so much we are willing and able to wish them into existence. Give me a break! Fortunately, that theory has been virtually eliminated with increased research and scientific study of the phenomena.

Our nerves are trying to do their job when limb removal occurs. They are constantly sending information on where our body is, what it is doing and what it is feeling in a variety of places all at once. They also serve as a valuable alarm system when sharp, heat, or pressure is becoming damaging to the body. But our nerves have also been damaged with the amputation so they are trying to heal and regroup. As with the phantom, the sensations we now feel may not correspond to reality.

Some of us really don't mind our phantom feeling. Mine fits right into my prosthesis and almost fools me into thinking that I have two legs.

The group, Pearl Jam, sang in their song, "Black, Red, Yellow", about phantom pain being all that's left of an amputated leg.[14]

Perhaps that's better than no feeling at all.

12 DOCTORS HAVE FEELINGS TOO

When we consider the emotions connected with an amputation, it is important to realize that all who are in close contact with the patient will also experience some feelings about it. That includes the health care team and, especially, the surgeon.

Research for this chapter included interviewing several surgeons; specifically those who specialize in vascular [blood vessel] problems and orthopaedics [bones]. These are typically the doctors who are called upon to do amputations. Also, over the course of my hospital nursing career, I informally communicated with many surgeons on this topic.

Salvage Preferred

All physicians prefer to save limbs rather than remove them. That's what they went to school for. They would much rather repair any damage, if at all possible, than amputate. The common theme I hear is, "Always err on the side of saving a limb." Understandably, most of us prefer that they think that way. Certainly removal can be done later, if needed, but an amputation is obviously irreversible.

Because of the finality of it, the pressure is on for the doctor and patient, to not be too hasty but to consider all options carefully. Sometimes the options are clearly limited. When the limb is crushed or gone, or the tumor is threatening life, or gas gangrene has set in; hard decisions need to be made quickly. At times like this a doctor with specialized experience in these cases can be a great asset. As one person stated, "It helps if your doctor has some gray hair." Everyone wants to feel that the amputation was done only because it was necessary and the involvement of an experienced specialist can provide that confidence. Several specialists are even better.

Destructive vs. Reconstructive

One of the reasons that surgeons don't want to do amputations is because it appears to be destructive. There is a visible gap where the extremity used to be. Removing other diseased or dysfunctional *internal* parts does not appear to have the same impact on either the surgeon or patient because of their lack of visibility. For example, removing a gallbladder, spleen, or even a uterus, leaves little more than an external scar, if that. However, there certainly can still be associated emotions, especially with the uterus removal.

In 1993, I did an extensive interview with Dr. Ernest Burgess. This orthopaedic surgeon received an international reputation as an expert in amputations as well as other orthopaedic surgery. His expertise began during World War II. Dr. Burgess shared that his enthusiasm for amputation surgery was fueled by his sincere belief that an appropriate amputation is actually *constructive surgery*. The removal of a severely damaged or diseased limb not only keeps the person alive, it usually aids in regaining good health and mobility again.

If done well, the surgeon reconstructs the end of the limb to wear an intimately fitting piece of advanced technology that can allow the person to bear weight. Regarding the leg, Dr. Burgess visualized that he was reconstructing the 'foot' at whatever level needed and that the prosthesis then became the extended 'boot' for that person to ambulate on. He stressed the careful handling and reattachment of the muscle, tendons and ligaments, with full knowledge of the desired weight bearing areas for ideal prosthetic use. Dr. Burgess truly became a creative plastic surgeon as he rebuilt the remainder of the limb for maximum durability and minimal discomfort.

When asked about the destructive nature that some of his peers saw in amputation, Dr Burgess replied, "All surgery in destructive."[15] This is a good point to ponder. Indeed, healthy tissue needs to be cut to even get *at* the problem area of the body. Blood is lost and tissue surrounding the problem is damaged to allow a healthy base for healing. So, in the end, the doctor and patient allow limited destruction to provide healthy reconstruction.

Quality of Life

Many experienced surgeons have come to a similar conclusion. With the first goal being salvage, the ultimate goal is survival, and from there, quality life. When the doctor takes the time to get to know the patient and for him to get to know the doctor, a positive first step is taken. Then as the patient recovers, the doctor does well to maintain caring communication. As life is reestablished, beyond just wound healing, the doctor will see that a timely, well-done amputation can return the person to a satisfying, productive life.

There is a warm satisfaction that comes with extending the life of a limb. Peers are impressed, and the patient and family are overjoyed that it was saved. Even the media steps up and describes how a disastrous injury was remedied by great medical intervention. But it doesn't always end well.

Once I heard a vascular surgeon share, at a medical conference, about saving a nearly destroyed limb. "Limb salvage can be kind of like peeing in your pants. At first it kind of makes you feel warm all over. But pretty soon you're not so sure you did the right thing."[16]

If the surgery is successful and heals well the physician may be pleased. However, perhaps, it doesn't feel like a success to the patient who lives with constant pain and a lack of function. One man fell from a sixth-floor platform while washing windows.

He shattered both feet and legs when he landed on them. Two years later he told me, as he hobbled into my office on his crutches, "They say I am lucky to still have my legs. But I don't feel so lucky."

Another older woman with blood vessel problems underwent multiple surgeries to keep blood flowing to a dying foot. "Of course, I want to keep my foot. But mostly I just want to go home and get my life going again. I want to live in my house, see my dog, cook my own dinner and drive my car…"It's one thing to advise limb verses life. It's extremely hard for the doctor to recommend limb verses independence. There always seems to be another procedure available, and with it, a glimmer of hope that this will be the one to keep our limbs and have a life.

Emotional Connection

One of the most positive doctor-patient relationships can evolve with an amputation. While the amputee has just experienced a most devastating loss, he appreciates:

- The surgeon who did a hard thing but the right thing.
- The surgeon who sat (not stood) at his bedside, taking precious time to explain why removal was being advised or necessary.
- The surgeon who followed him afterward; through healing, therapy, prosthetic fitting and into life.
- The surgeon who cared.

Not all surgeons provide this level of involvement, but when they do, it becomes a satisfying, growing experience for them and the patient.

The doctors interviewed described a need to be focused and clear-thinking when doing the surgery. Their emotions cannot, and should not interfere with the work being done. Nonetheless, emotion can be felt and shown before and after the procedure. Their caring may be demonstrated in compassionate words, time, or even tears.

A missionary doctor shared that he cared for another missionaries' small child once in a remote place. Careful surgery, done several times, would not heal. The sutures just fell out as the wound came open and the child eventually died. The doctor wept with the family. Decades later the former missionaries invited him to speak at their church in the United States. He was reluctant and not sure how they felt about the tragedy even now. He went and was overwhelmed when he was introduced as 'the doctor who cried with us when our precious girl died.' No blame and no fault. He came to see the truth of the statement, 'Doctors treat, God heals'. He had provided the best treatment he knew and the family was grateful.

Of course, it's a balance. As one doctor said, "The patient or family doesn't want a crybaby surgeon. But they don't want one who is cold or indifferent either."

When there is not a relationship between the doctor and patient, many inaccurate perceptions can emerge. Confidence may be eroded. The patient may feel that the doctor doesn't really care. A variety of thoughts may be expressed:
- He was in a hurry.
- He did the easy thing.
- Saving money was all he cared about.
- He knew I was on welfare.
- He was prejudiced against my being Indian or Polish or…
- I'm going to sue.

Establishing a caring relationship with a patient is always worth the investment, especially with an amputation.

Hard Cases

The hardest cases for doctors are typically the younger ones. No one wants to see an innocent child have to deal with such a big loss as an amputation. Many are preventable as with lawn mower injuries.

If the doctor has a child of similar age it's hard not to see their own child as they carry out the necessary surgery.

Bone tumors are also most difficult. A healthy looking limb, or a portion thereof, may need to be removed because of the deadly disease lying underneath.

One doctor described the agony of removing the leg of a healthy-looking eighteen-year-old woman. "She had two beautiful legs. It felt criminal to cut one away. I had to focus on the tumor to do it at all."

Another surgeon spoke of a young football player under his care. "He thought it was a bad knee injury but there was a deadly tumor lurking inside. He was so muscular and young. Doing the right thing for him was hard."

There is obviously a clearer sense of positive impact when removing a putrid, deformed, blackened foot. Especially on someone who has more years behind them than ahead. The hard part here is to take enough of the limb to allow it to heal quickly. The effort to save as much as possible sometimes causes the surgeon to remove the dead tissue at a level that also has limited blood supply. To get the person out of the hospital and back to life, it is important to remove up to a healthy level of blood circulation. Being too conservative risks non-healing, more surgery, extended hospital stays and sometimes even death.

The surgeon's best approach is to closely follow the patient before and after the procedure. Again they provide themselves the privilege of a relationship with the patient and the often positive outcome of having a damaged/diseased limb removed. The person can then move on to a life of quality, independence and function. He knows that it was the surgeon who provided the first intervention in making this all possible.

13 MONEY – THE BOTTOM LINE

When the impact of limb loss strikes the cost issues and concerns can rise to the top. For many of us, money is often a primary daily concern anyway. Now the person with a fresh amputation is struck with serious thoughts. *Is this covered by insurance? Can I afford what is happening to me? Can my family afford it?*

Home Management and Care of Others

Not everyone is involved in outside employment but the work they do is valuable to keeping a home organized, clean and functioning and caring for the people that live there. When the home manager/caregiver is dealing with a limb loss, the entire family faces upheaval and tremendous expense can be incurred in trying to replace her or him. Some people in this circumstance are able to enlist a family member (grandparent, aunt, etc.) to cover for basic childcare, at least temporarily. Others have found church and extended community helpful. Unfortunately, many people don't have family nearby, or, if they do, they have jobs, health issues or other barriers to stepping in to help. To actually pay for the twenty-four-hour services of a homemaker/parent/caregiver can be cost prohibitive.

Insurance

Medical insurance, or the lack thereof, can be an

overwhelming concern. Even if the surgery and hospital costs are covered, will the artificial limb be provided? Especially disturbing is the information that a prosthesis can cost as much as a new car, or more. Many insurance policies cover only one prosthesis per lifetime or merely a fraction of their full cost.

One family had a small but growing restaurant. The wife was the main cook and manager. Due to exorbitant premiums, they chose to have limited medical coverage. This did not cover prosthetics or other 'durable medical equipment' like crutches, wheelchairs, and bathtub support bars. It proved to be a disaster when she was in a car wreck and needed a leg amputation. Even though the community rallied with a fundraiser and varied support, she was not able to do the demanding work of keeping the business running during her recovery and they had to close their beloved home-style restaurant.

Cost to Family

More immediate thoughts also include lost wages of the patient or those of family members who choose to be at our side. Perhaps the medical care we are receiving is a long distance from family and the commute is costly. "My wife has taken time off work and has expenses of gas, parking, food and hotel as she drives from two states away to be with me." reported one man from Montana.

It seems to be the rare individual who has no money concerns during recovery from limb loss. Most of us have very real thoughts of paying today's bills and the overwhelming fears of dealing with future expenses.

Employment

There are a few people whose ability to be productive is not affected to a great degree by an amputation. One fellow I recall was a writer and was not concerned at all about his work even with both lower legs amputated. Another was a businessman who spent most of his time at a desk so he quickly returned to work in a wheelchair as his leg amputation healed.

The problem arises for the person who relies on the mobility, balance, strength and skill of his body to make a living. The logger, construction worker, longshoreman, farmer or skilled tradesman, often has many justifiable concerns about his future. It is one thing to still be able to build a house or cut down trees but is it now a reasonable way to make a living? "I don't want to slow the rest of the crew down or be unsafe for them or me in the process," stated one forty-two-year old roofer. "I know I will need to make some changes."

Many people in physical jobs enjoy working with their body and being out of doors. The idea of working at a desk is abhorrent to some. As I listen to and counsel such people, I occasionally will suggest that they return to their work if their employer is supportive, and see how it goes. But they should always to keep in mind that a change may be a wise part of their future. Many will admit that their job, because of the physical demands, was not one that they planned to stay with indefinitely anyway.

Perhaps there are adaptations that can be made at work to be less demanding physically. In the work world they often refer to it as light duty. In my early years as a nurse, I experienced pain and skin problems on my stump as I attempted to work on my feet for eight hours, lifting, turning and transporting patients. As mentioned previously, I was grateful when my employer assigned me to the newborn nursery to lift these much lighter patients and sit with them or hold them as part of my work. Eventually I transferred to the night shift on a regular ward which allowed some sitting time for charting, ordering supplies and other documentation type chores.

Many people I know, like the middle aged roofer, have happily shifted within their jobs to quality control, getting bids, giving estimates or providing general management. That works well for the person who enjoys their work and has significant experience. However, not everyone feels that way about their work.

Some never really liked their job anyway but it bought groceries. The responsibilities of life kept them from making a change – until now. One immigrant from Fiji worked in a factory building furniture and was never real comfortable working around the dangerous machinery. He certainly didn't want to return to it now after losing an arm caught in a conveyor system.

This tragedy can become an opportunity as they step out and start the small business that was always in the back of their mind or return to school to develop their minds more than their backs. The young Fijian man above went to school to become a property assessor and obtained a government office job. Once again he could provide for his wife and growing family. How good it feels to eventually earn a paycheck and become productive, especially with a limb or two missing.

It seems that the biggest changes required are in the most physical jobs. These jobs are hard work for people that are young and totally healthy. Fortunately, one of the joys of being human is how versatile we can be with our body, mind and talents. We need to be willing to change but it can be done. An animal that loses a limb is out of commission for the most part, especially in the wild. But we humans can go another direction with our productivity as we study, learn to use our mind more, operate high tech equipment, or develop latent skills and talents.

Professional Performers

On this same note are the people who have become professional athletes or high-level performers. They may still have fun with friends or their kids in a game of tag football but playing in the National Football League with a missing limb is a whole different level. It is something I would not recommend. The basketball player may not be able to earn a living, as before, in his sport but he can still play recreationally with friends and family.

Dancing with friends or your spouse may work fine but performing in a professional ballet is a two-legged project. In most cases these people I'm referring to are still athletes or dancers but re-achieving the level they once had with a body possessing less original equipment can be frustrating, if not futile.

The goal to seek in this situation is not the high performance but rather maintaining the identity of being an athlete, entertainer, dancer, musician, artist, etc. Like the artist that paints with the brush in her teeth, we become very aware that our talent is not in our hands but in our mind.

Occasionally our uniqueness becomes a plus as we market ourselves to the world. One young man was able to earn income by his extreme skiing; then he was hit by a car as he was helping-load a truck. His leg was removed above the knee and that familiar lament was heard "I'll never ski again." However, he recovered and chose to not only ski but to resume his extreme skiing as a one-legged athlete. Surprisingly to him, the endorsements and sponsors were even more interested in his unique approach.

The moral is, don't let your amputation take more of you than necessary. Be prepared to make some changes. Try doing what you did without the limb. Be a one-armed drummer or a one-legged cyclist. If that isn't satisfactory then make adaptations to your sport, music, dancing or art. Adapt the musical instrument. Consider a high-energy or uniquely-made replacement limb. Technology is helping on all sides with this. As the old US Army slogan says, "Be all you can be."

14 FEELINGS ABOUT MY PROSTHESIS

Disappointment
So this is it..? This piece of lifeless material will replace a part of my flesh and bone. I feel sick to my stomach as I look it over, put it on and try to use it.

Many people are disappointed with the early artificial limb. The pain of saying goodbye to our precious body part is still fresh. We are in the middle of our grief and this is the replacement for warm, sensitive, useful flesh? It's so inhuman, weird looking, and just, well, artificial.

It's heavy, clunky, ugly and not much at all like a real limb. Sometimes it seems better to have the first prosthesis just left in the uncovered state with the metal pylon (pipe) and mechanical parts all showing. It looks obviously artificial and that's just the way it is. Besides, it makes all the early fitting adjustments that much simpler. The prosthetist [the one who makes a replacement body part] doesn't have to rip off the outside cover every time some little change is needed. It does make our challenge more visible to others. When we limp or struggle to keep up, the world is usually more patient with us. The problem is we want so bad to look 'normal' again. We don't want to have people take second or subtle looks as we wheel, crutch, or limp past.

Prosthetist

Speaking of the prosthetist, most of us had never even heard the word before. We often spend many months in their care before we can even say their title correctly. The word itself sounds like a woman who earns money working the night shift out on the streets. But, seriously, I personally came to admire this person for the very challenging job they had of trying to replace my precious body part.

The best prosthetists are the ones who join up with us to become a team member in this project. They are taking on a monumental endeavor to make a limb that is comfortable, durable, reliable, functional, and *looks like the limb it replaces*. There are always tradeoffs. We can't have all of this in our limb but with much persistence and effort we may get most.

One of my best prosthetists asked me, before starting, "What would you like in this limb?" He spent time getting to know me and letting me know how he was going to work on making what I needed. Essentially, he demonstrated that he cared.

In my opinion, the worst prosthetists are those who treat you like you are on an assembly line. They have done this before and know what you need. If you're not happy with it, well, "You just need to accept that you're an amputee now." This is what you get.

The First Prosthetic

In the beginning, the socket part of the artificial limb that fits snugly over the remaining part of our body is bigger than it ultimately will be. The swelling from the surgery will take several months or even a year to decrease. Normal shrinkage of the muscle in the stump will also occur. In the beginning it always looks and feels much bigger than our other leg. Any previous clothes that fit snugly at the knee or thigh, now strain to stretch over the prosthesis. Some won't even go on over it. We've lost a part of our body and now we need to part with some previous clothing that was also well liked, comfortable and/or attractive. The forced changes and losses keep mounting.

One young woman was not pleased but put on her new prosthesis and covered it carefully with a heavy nylon-type stocking. With new shoes on she hurried over to her girlfriends' house on crutches to demonstrate her new leg. Her friend tried to be sensitive but couldn't hide her surprise as she honestly remarked "It's so big. Will they be able to make it look more like your other leg?"

So even if you try and overlook and accept the unattractive early stage of the limb replacement, other people may not know how to.

Reality

Waking up during those early months is so hard. How we long to rub our feet together as we had for so many years, to simply scratch our ankle with our other toes. A quick glance at the bed and the flat area where a limb once was, confirms that this isn't just a nightmare. Our limb is really gone and it isn't coming back. Instead we now have this appliance to replace it and there it sits, or stands, by our bed. "I couldn't bear waking up and looking at this thing, so for several days I hid it behind the nightstand. I could reach it but didn't have to look at it first thing," remarked one person.

There seems to be something almost spooky about an artificial limb. It resembles a body part laying or standing there in your bedroom. Of course, it's *supposed* to resemble a body part. But there's something weird about that; even if it's a wig on your dresser or a set of dentures in a cup. They aren't extra adornment but actual body part substitutes. How weird is that? Also, who wants to wake up to see parts of themselves waiting close by to be put back on? Of course, it's worse to *not* have replacement parts to fill in our gaps, but that's another issue.

If you think you can probably get used to waking to a limb or other part near the bed, you start to consider other folks who may need to get used to it. First your spouse; how does she feel about it? She needs time to get used to how it looks, where it sits and waking up to it too. It's important to have a conversation about the whole issue and consider her feelings and process of emotional adjustment also.

And what about camping out? Do you keep the limb in the sleeping bag so the rest of the people on the wilderness raft trip aren't startled to see it lying outside? Or worse, do you actually try to sleep with your prosthesis on? That can be a major discomfort. I've tried it. A person may as well sleep with their hiking boots on. It is not a good idea.

Sometimes we may stay over at a relative's or share a hotel room at a conference. Once I roomed with a lady I had never met at a women's retreat. I just told her right up front that this fake limb is what I live with and she may see it by the bed or hear me putting it on at night to go to the bathroom. She turned out to be a physical therapist and was totally intrigued and, impressed by it all.

Clothing Alterations

With or without our prosthesis, even the simple things of getting dressed become more complex. It now takes more time and planning. Eventually it becomes a common part of our life but at first it feels like it takes so much more time even though it's usually only a few minutes. One elderly gentleman remarked with humor, "We don't get dressed, we get assembled."

Shoes and clothes are an early detail to work with. Should we just toss the fancy high heels? How about the flat, but so comfortable sandals, with no strap on the back or the cowboy boots that the prosthetic foot won't bend to fit into? Some shoes just aren't practical for safety and fit reasons. Other shoes are important to you for comfort or appearance. Maybe the shoes or boots have even become a part of your identity. If so, some alterations at the shoe repair shop may be in order. The cowboy boots can be altered with a zipper or even bought that way. Some now have lower heels and even laces. It's good to consider all the available options to minimize more losses.

Usually some extra shopping is required to find shoes for the prosthetic foot to fit well and look good. The process must include the comfort of our remaining foot. This is especially so for those with diabetes or circulation problems in their real foot. Fortunately some sandals and clogs have a heel strap which helps hold them on the prosthetic side. After all these years, shopping for shoes is still the one thing that can almost drive me to tears.

High heels are often an important issue to some of us females. In the beginning I wanted to wear high heels for my wedding and other dressy occasions. About two years after my injury, when the shrinking on my short leg had stabilized, I invested in a special high heeled leg. Her name was 'Lady' and I wore her for several years at certain times, including my wedding. She made feel and look more like a 'lady'. Ultimately, however, I found I couldn't walk as comfortably or as far in her. I traded her for a much lower stacked heel type foot which allows some dressier shoes than flats. Over time I have noticed that as we women mature we often pick more sensible styles anyway. Looks are sometimes bypassed for comfort and mileage.

Regarding clothes, the short skirts or shorts display the whole artificial set up. We may want to look normal so badly again that we decide to toss these items too. However, many people find that later, when they don't feel as sensitive, these clothes are ok. Other folks are comfortable in shorts from the beginning and almost enjoy the uniqueness of their appearance. And there's no denying that we are unique people.

Some of the looser fitting clothes are fine but the snug, form-fitting ones, especially at the joints, just don't do well. Not only do they display the ridges and other parts of the prosthesis, they actually destroy clothing, particularly at the joints (knee, hip, elbow, etc.). In the process of walking they can limit mobility as they bind with the clothing. It can all feel so frustrating. *I already lost my leg. I don't want to lose all the clothes and shoes that were part of my wardrobe and appearance too!* Besides, in the early days we usually don't have the energy or money to replace them all anyway. It becomes a process over time to select shoes and clothes that work with our revised body.

Comfort and Feel

At best, especially in the beginning, the prosthetic feels uncomfortable. It's heavy and tight. We're not used to having a piece of high tech equipment strapped firmly onto our body. It puts pressure on so many areas that we're not used to. These tissues were not made to fit snugly into a container and withstand our body weight and movement. But we're making it do it. Usually it's not all bad. It's probably like a person who never wears shoes and now is trying or required to or like a person getting used to contacts or dentures.

There can be outright pain in some spots but a good prosthetist is usually determined to eliminate that. Thank goodness. At least the pain should be minimized to a tolerable level of discomfort. If the fit is bad, just looking at the prosthesis can be painful. If every step hurts or we can't be comfortable even sitting with the limb, we may not even choose to wear it.

Removal of all discomfort is sometimes not possible by the prosthetist. In my early years as an amputee, there was one bony prominence on the stump that was impossible for the limb maker to work around. Ultimately, I returned to have the surgeon fine tune it. My surgeon had a different idea of what to do than what the prosthetist suggested. I went with what the prosthetist said because I knew that once the wound healed, I would never see the surgeon again. My limb maker would now be a part of my life.

The weight of the prosthesis is located solely around the socket and suspension area. If our remaining limb is shorter than ideal, it minimizes our ability at leveraging that weight. Like holding a hammer at the end of the handle it feels heavier than if we hold it at the center. If our remaining limb goes to mid-calf or mid-thigh, it becomes much easier to manipulate the prosthesis.

Since we have no control over the length of limb we are left with, it's an advantage when the prosthetics are made lighter. Fortunately, in recent years there have been some very positive changes in the heaviness of the prosthesis due to the replacement of old materials with light-weight, space-age types. Now instead of wood, leather, and steel, we have titanium, graphites, nylon, and carbon fiber. The newer material is typically lighter and more durable although a few people still prefer the more natural older materials that may conform to the body and 'breathe' better.

Reliability

For many of us this prosthetic leg will serve us fairly well. It will walk, fill out our clothes, stay upright, and even do some extra kicking, dancing, and running under our power and limited coordination. But there are times when it will catch on a rug, tip into a hole, or maybe even break and pull us down if we don't catch ourselves first. It can be downright embarrassing as we gracefully try to get up from the floor, hopefully without physical injuries. Actually, without a prosthesis we are vulnerable to trip and slip around even more with our crutches.

Assuming that we really aren't hurt when a fall like this occurs, it's handy to have a good sense of humor. In fact, it's a good idea to have a sense of humor about this whole amputation experience.

One fellow was in a theater lobby when his prosthetic ankle made a noticeable cracking sound as he went down. He quickly realized that the new ankle he was testing had given out. "Oh, I guess I broke my ankle," he said casually as he attempted to get up. A horrified lady at the counter said, "Oh, my! Should I call 911?" He gently assured her that this ankle needed no medical attention since it was not real flesh & bone. This information didn't seem to calm her much, though, as she tried to process it all. It still makes a funny story to share with friends.

Fortunately, unless we have other issues, most of us rarely fall. In the beginning it's more of a risk as we attempt to establish our balance and coordination with our appliance. Later we become wiser and more careful around new, wet or uneven territory. Slowing the pace, sometimes dramatically, can usually keep us upright. Ice and snow are tricky but they are for whole-bodied people too. Once I thought I would go down as I came down a steep Seattle street during a hail storm. I turned sideways like I was skiing but the hailstones kept moving me like little ball bearings. Somehow, I stayed upright anyway.

Finally, to add to our limb's reliability, we do well to keep duct or duck tape nearby, especially when traveling. Of course, we know that this item can get us through all kinds of temporary emergencies in life. Some people also carry an Allen wrench or hex key with them to secure the foot, if needed. Others will travel with a pair of crutches for a backup mobility system. Personally, I have rarely had need for either of the latter two but *always* have duct tape along. A prosthesis may break but won't usually fall completely apart. Once I fell on an icy sidewalk with a loud crash. I was sure my fake leg was now in pieces. But, no, the rest of me was bruised but the leg had nary a scratch.

Safety

An early concern has to do with safety. *What do I do if the house catches on fire at night and I need to get out fast? How do I grab clothes and a leg and get out the door? I can't forget the socks or liner as the leg is not wearable without them.* There are so many details to consider in this altered body. More than other people, we need to make a plan ahead of time about where the door is, have the limb and socks close, and be prepared to slip it on quick or hop or crawl outside with it in an emergency. When I travel I always check the hotel map for the nearest exit for this very purpose.

It's a known fact that muggers look for people along the street that look more vulnerable; older, handicapped, pregnant. They select someone that can't fight back, run fast or just looks more helpless. So if you wear a prosthesis, wear it with an air of confidence and ability, especially if it is conspicuous. If you need to travel in public in a wheelchair or on crutches try to go in daylight in well-traveled areas. It always feels better to have a friend along if I am on crutches.

Several men have commented that they don't feel as capable as the protector of their family following limb loss. Whether it's rushing to grab a stray toddler, defending their wife in a threatening situation or getting their family out of danger; they just don't feel as fast or as strong. This decreased coordination also provides a certain threat to their masculinity. Most men want to resume their role as protector and all that it entails. Using brains instead of brawn may be a better approach anyway. When possible, avoid risky places and people.

On that same note I have spoken to several wives of male amputees. Unlike the common role of the husband to check out suspicious noises at night, it is only logical for the wife to have that job since she doesn't have to 'get assembled' first. One lady laughed as she described how she takes a weapon along (broom, bat, etc.) as she goes alone to check what made a thump in the night.

Ongoing Adjustment

People have reported intense frustration in the early stages of prosthetic use. Some have thrown the limb across the room, down the stairs, or, even, out the window. Because of its being significantly expensive, they usually don't go farther than that in abusing it.

A less destructive way to cope with prosthetic frustration is humor, and lots of it. I have heard and read about so many stories where humor lightens the challenges.

One well-groomed, older gentleman shared that as he was riding on the bus once, and a middle aged woman sat beside him. He was wearing his full-length, old style, wooden prosthesis which was completely covered by his suit slacks. The woman accidentally bumped his leg. Startled by how solid it felt she rudely said, "What is that?" My friend calmly replied, "That, my dear, is a leg made out of the same thing as your head!"

Some people enjoy unique demonstrations with their prosthesis for unknowing observers. One boy turned the foot backwards to make tracks in the snow. He said he wanted to make sure no one followed him.

I knew a fisherman who enjoyed filleting his fish at the lake while others watched and stabbing the knife into his prosthetic thigh until he needed it again. A seamstress wasn't quite as dramatic, found that the foam cover on the leg made a handy pincushion.

Arm amputees seem to have fun with the hook device as they turn the meat on the barbeque or pull things out of the oven without a glove. There's a practical side to that too as long as it doesn't damage the prosthesis.

Of course it's hard to beat the pirate costume option for parties at certain times of the year. Either the hook hands or peg legs are quite dramatic looking. By adding an eye patch and/or a fake parrot on your shoulder you will come across looking unique. Once I wore a pirate costume with a peg leg as I gave out candy to the children on Halloween at my front door. I heard one of them comment as he walked away, "Did you see that lady? She had a toilet plunger on her leg! I wonder how she got it to stay on?"

Conclusion

Over time, and with a good fit, your artificial limb can feel less like a spooky invader and more like a friend. You feel less 'handicapped' with it because it enables you to look and function more like you used to. It's still a long shot from how your real limb looked and moved but it's way ahead of nothing at all.

One final comment on this topic is that many people do <u>not</u> have the privilege of dealing with a prosthesis early on, if at all. This may be due to the condition of their residual limb, their general health, their finances, or the country where they happen to live. Typically these folks don't experience many of the above emotions because they are so grateful to finally have a prosthesis that they don't struggle as much with its imperfections.

15 SUMMARY OF COPING WITH LIMB LOSS

At the beginning of this book we identified how massive the impact of limb loss is. Every aspect of our life is touched or totally changed by it. Occasionally it is changed for the better as we work to eliminate our irresponsible or destructive behavior. Let's review how to move through this amputation adjustment process.

Grief

We must give ourselves the **privilege of grieving** if we are to move forward. Our loss is profound, whether we realize it or not. We cry, talk, journal and utilize our creative skills to express our pain and sometimes share it with others. Keeping all our feelings inside is destructive. Avoiding reality with drugs, prescriptive or otherwise, is also destructive.

The appendix of this book contains a listing that I have compiled of ways to work through our grief *(What to do with Loss)* and another for helping someone else to grieve *(Helping Others with Loss)*. We are not on an easy road, to be sure. But it is truly character-building and holds many joyful surprises.

Support System

Getting through the transition of limb loss should not be attempted alone, although some have done it. It's easier if we make use of those who care. Ideally this incorporates our faith, our family and friends.

For me this began in prayer to my God who loves me and promised never to leave me. It included conversation with the family and friends that were there for me. It included crying with some of them.

Other support can also include professionals who are there to listen and encourage and provide wise counsel. Remember, this is a *big* project. It is not a sign of weakness to seek emotional support. It's a sign of good sense.

Support Group

As mentioned earlier, one of the best connections that can be made for recovery is meeting other people who have come through amputation, especially those who have done it successfully. Picture yourself being lost in the woods. Then you encounter someone who has found a path that will take you out of this confusing, unknown place. What a gift. Their path might not be the exact path you would have picked but it got them out and moving forward. Much can be learned as you listen to their experience – what worked and what didn't.

In the beginning, the more amputees you meet and converse with, the better. That's where a support group comes in. Some people you may be barely able to relate to, while others approach challenges like this much like you do. Most have some helpful experiences that you can learn from and apply to your own situation.

Information

There is a mountain of new information to be dealt with as we survive, deal with surgery, care for our wound, heal and move back to a productive life. We must first get our body systems working in a healthy fashion. Our lungs, blood circulation, stomach, bowels and every other part of our body have been impacted. If disease has brought all this on, we must consider what is needed to revive and protect a body that is already struggling. Our wound healing may take longer. Wearing a prosthetic may be delayed or not even advisable. A change in our lifestyle may be crucial to preserving the remaining leg. Knowing what to do and how to go about it is the first step. Actually carrying it out is the hard part.

There is a national organization called the Amputee Coalition of America (www.amputee-coalition.org), mentioned previously. This organization has a wealth of information available. They have magazines, books and a special booklet on new amputee information. They can even help you locate a support group or a trained amputee visitor in your area. There are some online posts which can be helpful if a face to face visit cannot be arranged. Keep in mind that, as with many subjects, people can say many things online but may not function or present themselves as well in person. In my opinion, a one on one visit by a trained visitor is ideal. The personal visit can be profoundly useful to family members who also have fears and many questions.

As a new amputee it is normal to feel lost, overwhelmed and even afraid. The health care people around you may attempt to encourage you with cases they've worked with or read about. But they haven't been through it! To meet a successful amputee at the right time is such joy. Here is a person who has found their way out of the woods and is eager to tell me where the trail is. A positive visit can instill the *hope* that we need so much.

Rebuilding Physically

Getting moving again will take significant effort, especially if your loss is a foot or leg, but includes arms as well. If an injury caused the loss it requires great recuperation of the body to heal and rebuilt its stamina. If disease is the cause, it can be an even greater challenge. The rest of your body continues to deal with a condition that claimed a part of it. There may be ongoing impact on other organs or other extremities. Usually we can't get back to where we were in total function but, over time, we establish a 'new normal' that can be quite satisfying. For example, hiking in the woods has always been a favorite activity of mine. I cannot hike as fast or as far as I once did but I am out there with my walking stick and so grateful for that.

The human body and mind doesn't do well with inactivity. Lying in bed may feel good for a couple of days but then we need to get back to business. This is especially so as the pain diminishes and our visitors move on with their lives. Yet we are cautioned to not move too fast. Our balance is out of order. Falling is a real danger. Wearing a prosthetic limb too soon and too much will result in skin breakdown and even more delays. Our world has become one of slow motion. Everything from getting dressed, to taking a shower, to carrying a cup of coffee, has become a deliberate effort. It can be beyond frustrating.

Working with physical therapy, ambulating with a wheelchair or crutches, and learning to use a prosthesis, may all be a part of what first needs to be accomplished. The activities of daily living (hygiene, cooking, shopping) are then taken on and sometimes done a little differently.

One of the best ways to get stronger again is to get back to the sports or activities we previously enjoyed: swimming, gardening, walking, golfing, skiing. Seek the things that have been enjoyable in your life. These things may require some adaptations but, for most of us, getting out there and doing an enjoyable activity under our own power is great satisfaction.

I've seen many people take on skiing after a limb loss and find a whole new sense of joy and inspiration. The two legged skier needs to adapt with firm boots, boards on their feet, and poles. We amputees adapt with a ski prosthesis or poles with short skis on the end. It's the same gravity that brings us all down the mountain. Like one fellow said after his first run on his remaining leg, "Hey, I think maybe I can go get a job now!"

Think Positive

Our mindset to get going again needs to be determined but realistic. One patient firmly announced that he was going to climb Mt. Rainier, the highest peak in Washington State. This was in spite of the fact that he had just lost both of his lower legs in a van accident. I encouraged him to walk up the steep hills of Seattle first. Not that he could never climb Mt. Rainier, but he was still flat on his back. The effort and energy required to walk on two artificial legs is profound. I knew that. But I also knew that it is not wise or caring to tell someone with a limb loss that they <u>couldn't</u> do something. Let him explore it and come to his own conclusions.

Focusing on what we still have and not what we've lost can help us move forward. Many things are different, slower and more deliberate. But we can usually figure out how to get them done. Like the fellow in the wheelchair said, with a grin, "I used to be able to do 10,000 things. Now I can only do 9,000." It's all in your perspective.

It's probably impossible, especially at first, to not compare how our life is now to how it was before. We must not dwell on it. This is how our life is now and, thank goodness, we are still alive. We can enjoy the people we love. We can enjoy the world around us. We can think and create. So much more is left than what we have lost.

And then there's the plus side. These kinds of experiences build character. We develop more compassion for others. We develop patience. We are strengthened by the very fact that we are a survivor. If we could survive this huge blow, we are surely able to withstand whatever else comes at us over time. We can begin to visualize real *hope* in our lives. Not 'I hope so' but the confidence that comes from being a survivor and overcomer. With this mindset we can be actually excited about our future and what it holds.

Humor

I can't stress humor enough. It can be found in everything, no matter how tragic and miserable it seems at first. Look for it. Hey, that athlete's foot skin problem is finally gone I can trim my toenails twice as fast as I used to. And out in the snow, I will only ever have just one cold foot!

My husband and I have two children, Troy and Tara. Once, after a shower I was putting my leg on and our then four-year-old son was watching. He had many questions. What's it made of? How does it stay on? Does it hurt?

Then I asked him, "Would you ever want one of these?"

He thought a moment and then firmly stated, "No...I'm going to be a *dad* when I grow up. Maybe Tara will want one. *She's* going to be a mom!"

And be sure to make use of puns. After all we want to start this journey by starting off on the right leg and end up standing on our own two feet. We'll join arm in arm with our fellow amputees as we reach out to give them a helping hand too. We want to get our foot back in the door of life without having to foot too much of the bill. It already feels like this whole experience is costing an arm and a leg. Life is good so let's be foot loose and fancy free. Let's kick up our heels and jump in with both feet. In the end let them say we towed the line and won hands down. I didn't let the other guy pull my leg or talk my leg off. I tried not to put my foot in my mouth or fill my hollow leg. So as we knuckle down to the work of it. We'll wash our hands of too much self-pity and move forward to the next leg of our journey. When our feet are on solid ground we will reach out to others on this path with open arms.

Utilize Necessary Available Benefits

When I first joined this community of people with a missing part or two I was unwilling to take the title of handicapped, disabled or whatever. I was still me and planned to stick with that. For ten years I refused to apply for a disabled parking permit. It felt like a sign on me and my car saying, "Yep, she's crippled all right."

It took a few rainstorms and icy sidewalks to convince me to rethink my approach. Walking the extra distance in bad weather and when my leg was hurting was no fun. Sometimes expensive closer parking was available but I was already spending more than the average person on nylons that ripped instantly, pants that wore out at the knee, shoes that needed reinforcement and repairs, etc. Initially my insurance did not cover artificial legs so I had to buy them for several thousand dollars. I finally decided that if society was going to offer me a closer and sometimes free parking spot, a discount on the bus, ferry or monorail, I was going to legitimately claim it.

Most days my leg does not hurt so I park farther away on purpose and rarely use the handicapped parking spots. I need the exercise, and besides I don't want to see someone with more extensive limitations than mine have to struggle more because I took the close-in parking spot.

As mentioned earlier, an area of benefit that I claimed was utilizing a state program that helped pay my schooling. It got me further educated in a field (nursing) that I was qualified to work in and allowed me to become self-supporting and independent. It turned out to be a valuable investment for the state as even now I continue to work and serve my community.

The thing we need to be careful about is claiming things we don't really need. Just because our insurance will cover a new prosthesis whenever we want it, we may not really need it. One lady I worked with got an unnecessary new limb often just because she was still covered on her ex-husband's policy. Another man had a work related injury and used his prosthesis for a tool to pound nails or submerged it in water for long periods. These kinds of abuse demonstrate an ungrateful and bitter attitude in us. Who needs it?

Some people receive an extraordinary financial settlement or are encouraged to take the title of 'disabled' to the point that they don't need to be employed. Employment is viewed as something to get out of and now they have a legitimate excuse. But in reality, working for our food and living has a psychological benefit. If we find ourselves in a place where we truly cannot be employed or don't have to work for these things we should be careful to do some meaningful work anyway for others and our own well-being.

A crippled mindset is a heavy burden.

Avoid Extensive Drug Use and Self-Pity

For many of us there is a great desire to withdraw as we grieve and attempt to cope with this overwhelming change to the body we once had. For a period of time this may be necessary and even healthy. But then we must move forward.

Some people find that the prescriptive medications for pain and depression help them escape emotionally. It all feels legitimate. After all it was a medical doctor that prescribed these drugs in response to our complaint of the pain and misery of it all. But it's now been months and we are afraid to let go of the fog of drugs and face our new reality. Our conspicuous loss makes it hard for the doctor and others to challenge our pain complaints and self-pity.

Others find that social drugs like alcohol, marijuana and even illicit drugs provide another nice escape. Notice these things are all just that, an escape. Staying drunk, stoned or just drugged into a stupor is not going to allow a person to move forward to the new life that awaits.

Reach Out to Others

After we've allowed some regroup time, we should seriously consider reaching out to others. Our own survival can be an encouragement to those who are also fresh into this unchosen life change. Helping others has a lot of positives, including pulling ourselves out of the self-pity mode. Helen Keller made a statement about getting stuck here. "Self-pity is our worst enemy and, if we yield to it, we can never do anything good in the world."

Probably the best reason for reaching out is that it puts some purpose into our own loss. We have gained some 'experience' credentials. We can see this whole limb-loss journey from the other side of the hospital bed rails. We understand some of the impact of it all even though we are still far from having all the answers.

As mentioned before, attending support groups for

amputees and those at risk for limb loss is a great start. It's not easy to do at first. We didn't even qualify for this group such a short time ago. Our identity is making a shift in this area. As we step out to see how others are making it through this adjustment we may get encouragement, new information, or offer advice ourselves. How good it feels to be not alone in this whole project.

Later we might explore becoming a peer visitor to others. This isn't for everyone but there is professional training for this position through the American Coalition of Amputees.[vi] I highly recommend it. Without the guidelines the ACA provides, it is possible to make it harder for new amputees to adjust. We may make inappropriate comments about their doctor, prosthetist or general recovery. Worse, we may spend the whole visit talking about ourselves and not even listen to them.

An example is one well-meaning visitor who spent the time discussing the advantages of his new prosthesis. According to him, this was the best foot, ankle and knee joint available. The new amputee was advised to not only get this type of limb but to get it through his prosthetist, who was, of course, described as the best around. However, a connection had already been made to a local prosthetist for this person, and a limb was being made. The limb was different than the visitor's because of other injuries, general health and activity level. This was quite confusing to the person with the new amputation. The visitor would have done better to ask the person about their current situation and listen, instead of trying to promote his own recovery approach. It's similar to a vehicle. We don't all need or want the same type of transportation. The guy living on a ranch wants a sturdy four wheel drive, not the slick sports car of the city guy.

Like all people, each of us living with a missing limb, is a unique individual. The ideal recovery for one may not work at all for another. Having said that, this book has attempted to address some of the basic steps that help all of us move forward, in our own individual style.

At the end of this chapter is a list of things to do in helping ourselves adjust to the profound experience of limb loss. Over and over I have seen the truth of the last statement on this list. We will be changed by this loss whether we like it or not. We will become bitter or better. We can become bitter about what has happened to us; bitter about life, bitter toward others, bitter toward God or we can become better people; stronger because we are survivors and over-comers. We may become more compassionate toward others who also live with obvious loss or imperfections. We can laugh at the days to come because we have found humor in even this. If we can get through this, there is nothing that can hold us back.

Dealing with Loss

1. Remember you are not alone. Seek out others who have successfully survived this type of loss.

2. An emotional loss is just as much a wound as a cut or a broken bone. The greater the loss, the more time and effort you'll need to heal.

3. Get more rest. Pamper yourself.

4. Reflect on how you've made it through past losses. If your approach worked well, use it again. If not, come up with a better plan.

5. Talk with appropriate family and friends who also feel the loss.

6. Tears are the safety valve of the heart. Crying is healthy physically and emotionally.

7. Accept comforting from others.

8. Make use of your spiritual beliefs i.e.: God's love, scripture, spiritual leaders, prayer and church family.

9. Know your resources for help.

10. Allow time for active grieving. Reminisce on good times with the lost limb(or person). Use visual items such as photos, letters, gifts.

11. Write a eulogy, letter to or a journal about the lost limb (person). See poem at end of this list.

12. Recognize present realities i.e.: the pain and suffering has diminished.

13. Draw, paint, sculpt or sew a picture of your grief.

14. Be willing to let go of your pain, anger and guilt.

15. Indulge in uplifting music and humor. It's ok to laugh.

16. Anticipate a future reunion, as your faith allows.

17. Reach out to help others.

18. You <u>will</u> become bitter or better from this. Let it be a positive growing experience.

Helping Others through Loss

1. Be with them. Your presence is valuable.

2. Listen without judgment. Give the maximum of your attention and the minimum of your intention.

3. Let them talk, or not.

4. Say, "I'm sorry," and "I care."

5. Touch and hug as is appropriate for this person.

6. Let the person cry. You may even cry with them.

7. Respect their beliefs. Offer to pray with them if you and they are comfortable with that.

8. Encourage use of their support system: faith, family and friends.

9. Share, briefly, if you have successfully survived a similar loss. How have they dealt with past losses? Did it work for them?

10. Their experience is unique. NEVER imply that you 'know exactly how they feel' even if you have had the same type of loss.

11. Anticipate what they need and provide it. Offer to do specific things (cooking, child care, cleaning, transportation, shopping, home or car repair, etc.).

12. Support their need for humor. Laugh with them.

Footstone

As insignificant as a foot may seem,
To be without one is for many a dream.

Here lies a foot the reason is known
Oh it's not all that bad for it was full grown.

It ran and it danced, it swam and it biked
It even walked through a meadow for which it had hiked.

It has since been replaced by a mechanical part
But know it will always have a place in my heart.

by Angela Hesler

March 9, 1999

Used by permission

Glossary of Terms Related to Amputation

Amputee -- A person who has had a limb, limbs, or a portion thereof, cut off (amputated).

Circulation -- Blood flow through the body. The movement of blood out of and back to the heart through the arteries and veins.

Dissupport--To provide help or comfort to a destructive degree. An example is when family treats a patient like he is helpless rather than allowing him to do what he is able to.

External Fixator --A metal framework that is outside the body but secured through the flesh to bones and holds them in place while they heal.

Fracture --A break in a bone.

Limb Difference--An arm or leg that is not fully intact due to birth, injury or disease.

Limb Salvage -- Efforts required to save an arm or leg or portion thereof.

Occupational Therapy --The teaching of how to perform activities of daily living as independently as possible, or to maximize independence in the case of disability.

Orthopaedics-- The medical specialty that focuses on injuries and diseases of the body's musculoskeletal system. It includes bones, joints ligaments tendons, muscles, and nerves. May correctly be spelled orthopaedics (British form) or orthopedics (Americanized version).

Outriggers--Ski poles with very short ski tips on the bottom end used to balance and maneuver while skiing.

Pin Sites--The openings in the skin where the metal fixator enters to secure itself to the bone.

Prosthetic--Item that serves as an artificial substitute for a body part like a limb, eye, or tooth.

Prosthetist (pros'-thi-tist)--A person who is involved in the science and art of prosthetics; one who designs and fits artificial limbs.

Pylon--A rigid tube between the temporary cast or socket of the prosthetic to the knee unit or foot that provides a weight bearing support shaft for the prosthesis.

Social Worker--A professional who assists with hospital discharge by coordinating access to needed services and organizations. Generally prepares a person for family and community life.

Terminal Device--An attachment to the wrist unit of an artificial arm prosthesis that provides some aspect of hand function like grasping and releasing.

Endnotes

1. Limb Loss Resource Center; Limb Loss Statistics: Amputee Coalition of America, 2014.

2. Wright-Parker, Jennie, RN,: Seven Stages of Grief: www.Recover-from-grief.com, 2004.

3. Mitchell, Margaret, <u>Gone With the Wind</u> , 1939. www.goodreads.com//quotes

4. Viscardi, Henry Jr. , <u>Give Us the Tools</u>, Erikson-Taplinger, 1959.

5. Amputee Coalition of America, Facebook post -

    https//:www.facebook.com/Amputee USA

6. Clark, James and Malchow, Dee. "Avoiding Errors in Limb Salvage Decisions", Orthopaedic Review. Vol. Xiii, No. 11:47-55, April, 1984.

7. Hansen, S.T.: Editorial: "The Type III C Tibial Fracture: Salvage or Amputation", Journal of Bone & Joint Surgery. 69-A:799-800, 1987.

8. Kohl, S: "The Process of Psychological Adaptation to Traumatic Limb Loss", in Krueger, D.W., Emotional Rehabilitation of Physical Trauma & Disability. New York. SP Medical & Scientific Books, pp. 113 - 148, 1984.

9. Jones, Susan: Harris Poll; December, 2013. http://cnsnews.com/news/article/susan-jones/poll-americans-belief-god-strong-declining

10. English Standard Bible: Romans 5:8; I John 4:16; Hebrews 13:5

11. Strohl, Daniel: Lost & Found; "Re: Chocolatier's Caddy". Hemmings Classic Car #86, November, 2011.

12. Legend, John and Gad, Toby: "All of Me"; Love in the Future, Album, 2013.

13. Hansel, Tim: You Gotta Keep Dancing, 1979. https://www.goodreads.com/author/quotes/55301.Tim_Hansel

14. Pearl Jam: "Black, Red, Yellow", written by Stone Gossard, Eddie Vedder, Jeff Ament, Mike McCready. Released 1996.

15. Burgess, Ernest M., MD: Quote used by permission.

16. Malone, James M. MD: Quote used by permission.

Made in the USA
San Bernardino, CA
28 October 2015